Current Topics in Microbiology and Immunology

234

Editors

R.W. Compans, Atlanta/Georgia
M. Cooper, Birmingham/Alabama
J.M. Hogle, Boston/Massachusetts · Y. Ito, Kyoto
H. Koprowski, Philadelphia/Pennsylvania · F. Melchers, Basel
M. Oldstone, La Jolla/California · S. Olsnes, Oslo
M. Potter, Bethesda/Maryland · H. Saedler, Cologne
P.K. Vogt, La Jolla/California · H. Wagner, Munich

Springer
Berlin
Heidelberg
New York
Barcelona
Budapest
Hong Kong
London
Milan
Paris
Santa Clara
Singapore
Tokyo

Clinical Applications of Immunotoxins

Edited by A.E. Frankel

With 16 Figures and 11 Tables

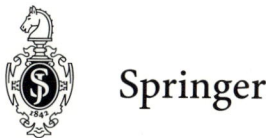 Springer

Arthur E. FRANKEL, M.D.
Associate Professor of Medicine
Medical University of South Carolina
Hollings Cancer Center
171 Ashley Avenue
Charleston, SC 29425-2850
USA

Cover Illustration: Pictured here are molecular models of targeted toxins. The ribbons are alpha carbon backbones of the following targeted toxins in clinical trials: a) upper left is DAB389IL2; b) lower left is LMB-7; c) right is anti CD19-bR. Green represents binding domains. Yellow represents enzymatic domains. Red is blocked Ricin B chain.

Cover Design: design & production GmbH, Heidelberg

ISSN 0070-217X
ISBN 3-540-64097-5 Springer-Verlag Berlin Heidelberg New York

This work is subject to copyright. All rights are reserved, whether the whole or part of the material is concerned, specifically the rights of translation, reprinting, reuse of illustrations, recitation, broadcasting, reproduction on microfilm or in any other way, and storage in data banks. Duplication of this publication or parts thereof is permitted only under the provisions of the German Copyright Law of September 9, 1965, in its current version, and permission for use must always be obtained from Springer-Verlag. Violations are liable for prosecution under the German Copyright Law.

© Springer-Verlag Berlin Heidelberg 1998
Library of Congress Catalog Card Number 15-12910
Printed in Germany

The use of general descriptive names, registered names, trademarks, etc. in this publication does not imply, even in the absence of a specific statement, that such names are exempt from the relevant protective laws and regulations and therefore free for general use.

Product liability: The publishers cannot guarantee the accuracy of any information about dosage and application contained in this book. In every individual case the user must check such information by consulting other relevant literature.

Typesetting: Scientific Publishing Services (P) Ltd, Madras

SPIN: 10498108   27/3020 – 5 4 3 2 1 0 – Printed on acid-free paper

Dedicated to my supportive, understanding wife–Jill, daughter–Rebeeca and son–Ian

List of Contents

D. FitzGerald, I. Pastan, and J. Robertus
Introduction 1

A. Engert, E.A. Sausville, and E. Vitetta
The Emerging Role of Ricin A-Chain Immunotoxins
in Leukemia and Lymphoma. 13

J.E. O'Toole, D. Esseltine, T.J. Lynch, J.M. Lambert,
and M.L. Grossbard
Clinical Trials with Blocked Ricin Immunotoxins 35

D.J. Flavell
Saporin Immunotoxins 57

F.M. Foss, M.N. Saleh, J.G. Krueger, J.C. Nichols,
and J.R. Murphy
Diphtheria Toxin Fusion Proteins 63

L.H. Pai and I. Pastan
Clinical Trials with Psedomonas Exotoxin Immunotoxins 83

E.H. Oldfield and R.J. Youle
Immunotoxins for Brain Tumor Therapy 97

A.E. Frankel and M.C. Willingham
Conclusions 115

Subject Index 121

List of Contributors

(Their addresses can be found at the beginning of their respective chapters.)

ENGERT, A	13	NICHOLS, J.C.	63
ESSELTINE, D.	35	O'TOOLE, J.E.	35
FITZGERALD, D.	1	OLDFIELD, E.H.	97
FLAVELL, D.J.	57	PAI, L.H.	83
FOSS, F.M.	63	PASTAN, I.	1, 83
FRANKEL, A.E.	115	ROBERTUS, J.	1
GROSSBARD, M.L.	35	SALEH, M.N.	63
KRUEGER, J.G.	63	SAUSVILLE, E.A.	13
LAMBERT, J.M.	35	VITETTA, E.	13
LYNCH, T.J.	35	WILLINGHAM, M.C.	115
MURPHY, J.R.	63	YOULE, R.J.	97

Introduction

D. FitzGerald[1], I. Pastan[1], and J. Robertus[2]

1	Introduction	1
2	Toxin Structure-Function Properties	2
2.1	Functions	2
2.2	Binding	3
3	Intracellular Processing – Cleavage and Reduction	4
3.1	Cytosolic Activity	5
4	Immunotoxin Design and Testing	6
5	Conclusion	8
References		8

1 Introduction

While various treatment approaches for cancer include reversal of the transformed phenotype, stimulation of immune responses, inhibition of metastatic spread and deprivation of key nutrients, the goal of immunotoxin treatment is the direct killing of malignant cells. Because they are enzymatic proteins that act catalytically to kill cells, bacterial and plant toxins are often employed as the cell-killing component of immunotoxins. Here we provide background information into the structure-function relationships of toxins and discuss how they can be combined with cell-binding antibodies or other ligands to generate immunotoxins.

Bacterial and plant toxins (e.g., diphtheria toxin, *Pseudomonas* exotoxin and ricin) are among the most toxic substances known. However, because they bind to cell surface receptors that are present on most normal cells, unmodified toxins are generally useless as anti-cancer agents. To convert toxins into more selective agents, their binding domains are either eliminated or disabled and replaced with cell-binding antibodies that are tumor-selective. Initially, immunotoxins were made by joining a modified toxin to an antibody molecule using chemical cross-linking

[1] Laboratory of Molecular Biology, Division of Basic Sciences, National Cancer Institute, NIH, Bldg 37/4E16, Bethesda, MD 20892, USA
[2] Department of Chemistry and Biochemistry, The University of Texas at Austin, Welch Hall 5.266 A, Austin, TX 78712-1167, USA

agents. More recently, gene fusion technology has been employed to generate recombinant immunotoxins. "Recombinant" usually (but not always – see CHEN et al. 1997) signifies that molecules have been expressed in *E. coli*.

Bacterial toxins such as DT and PE are single chain proteins that are secreted from bacterial cells into the surrounding media. These toxins were studied originally because of the tissue damage associated with certain bacterial infections of humans. Later it was appreciated that this destructive activity could be harnessed and redirected to kill cancer cells.

Plants also make a number of very toxic proteins. Toxins that cause damage to mammalian ribosomes, called ribosome inactivating proteins or RIPs, are frequently utilized in immunotoxin construction. RIPs are divided into two main classes. Type 1 RIPs are single chain proteins of approximately 30kDa that lack intrinsic cell binding activity and are exemplified by such toxins as pokeweed antiviral protein (PAP) and gelonin. Type 2 RIPs are heterodimers consisting of an enzymatically active domain, or A chain, linked by a disulfide bond to a binding domain, or B, chain. Ricin and abrin are two well known examples of this class of plant toxin.

2 Toxin Structure-Function Properties

2.1 Functions

The genes for DT, PE and ricin have been cloned and sequenced (GRAY et al. 1984; GREENFIELD et al. 1983; LAMB et al. 1985). DT is encoded by a transducing β-phage that infects *Corynebacterium diphtheriae*, PE is encoded from the chromosome of *Pseudomonas aeruginosa* and ricin is expressed in germinating castor beans. Structural data are available from protein crystals of each toxin (ALLURED et al. 1986; BENNETT and EISENBERG 1994; CHOE et al. 1992; KATZIN et al. 1991; LI et al., 1996; MONTFORT et al. 1987; RUTENBER and ROBERTUS 1991; WEISS et al. 1995) – see below. A combination of biochemical and cell biology studies have shown that these proteins have three signature functions: binding, translocation and catalysis (Fig. 1). While the binding and catalytic domains of each toxin have been assigned to specific structural elements, the structures that mediate translocation have been more difficult to define. With the exception of diphtheria toxin, in which translocation has been attributed to the action of two α-helical structures (KAUL et al. 1996), there is scant information regarding the location or mechanism of translocation.

Because full-length toxins usually do not reach the cytosol, processing steps that produce enzymatically active toxin fragments need to be considered. Once produced, it is these fragments that translocate to the cytosol and catalytically shut down protein synthesis. On route to the cytosol, toxins are subjected to limited proteolysis but must avoid complete degradation both by lysosomal enzymes and,

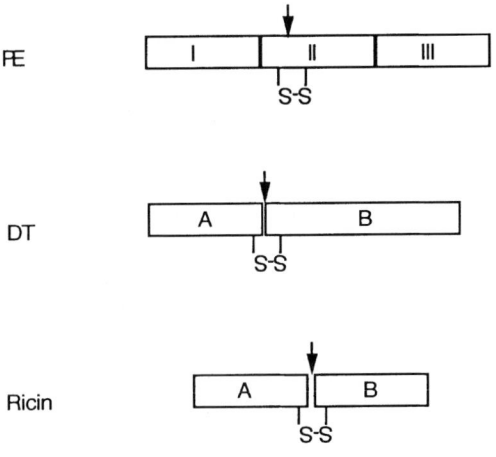

Fig. 1. Toxin structure-function. Toxins are composed of three structural domains that function to promote binding, translocation and enzymatic inactivation of protein synthesis

once in the cytosol, by proteasomes. Lysosomal delivery is probably avoided by sequences in the toxin that guide its movement to specific organelles. For instance, DT is brought to acidic endosomes and from there translocates to the cytosol (LEMICHEZ et al. 1997). PE and ricin follow a retrograde pathway to the endoplasmic reticulum and translocate from this organelle (CHAUDHARY et al. 1990a; PELHAM et al. 1992; WALES et al. 1993). While translocation to the cytosol is a key feature of toxins (and some viral proteins) it remains a poorly understood phenomenon. Once in the cytosol, the active fragments of DT and PE ADP-ribosylate elongation factor 2 (COLLIER 1988), while ricin A chain and its plant toxin cousins have N-glycosidase activity and remove the sugar base from 28S ribosomal RNA (ENDO et al. 1987).

2.2 Binding

The binding domains for the bacterial and plant toxins have been located. For DT and ricin, binding sequences are located at the COOH-terminal portion of the proteins. In contrast, the NH_2-terminal domain of PE mediates binding. DT binds the heparin-binding, epidermal growth factor (EGF)-like growth factor precursor found on most mammalian cells but absent on rodent cells (NAGLICH et al. 1992a,b). PE binds to the α2-macroglobulin receptor (also known as the low density lipoprotein receptor-related protein, LRP) (FITZGERALD et al. 1995; KOUNNAS et al. 1992). Ricin B chain is a sugar-binding protein with a preference for galactosides (BAENZIGER and FIETE 1979). Many proteins and lipids on the surface of eukaryotic cells display galactosides. Ricin B chain has at least two galactose-binding sites each of which binds sugar with only modest avidity (ZENTZ et al. 1978). Evidence for the existence of a third functional binding site has been reported recently (FRANKEL et al. 1996; LAMBERT et al. 1991). When these sites work in concert, ricin binds quite tightly to cell surfaces, with association constants of near 10^{-8}M. Ricin B chain association with the target cell surface facilitates uptake by endocytosis and the toxin may be processed as it moves through various intracellular compartments prior to translocation across the membrane (SANDVIG et al. 1994).

Recent results from Soria et al. have indicated that type I RIPs and the A chains of type II RIPs may use the α2-macroglobulin receptor to gain entry to cells (CAVALLARO et al. 1995; CAVALLARO and SORIA 1995). While binding to this receptor is likely to be a low affinity interaction, it may contribute significantly to in vivo toxicity.

Removal of the endogenous toxin-binding domains produces proteins that are usually not toxic for intact cells. The subsequent acquisition of novel binding domains can then direct the toxin to specific target cells. In most, but not all, cases replacement binding domains restore toxicity and target cells are killed. In those cases in which this is not true, it is probable that the new binding domains direct intracellular trafficking to nonproductive organelles. In those instances in which replacement of the toxin-binding domain with an antibody produces an immunotoxin of poor cytotoxic activity, the retention of a mutant binding domain has been a tactic to produce effective immunotoxins. For PE, this has meant the use of PE4glu, a mutant form of the toxin with four basic residues in the binding domain changed to glutamic acid (CHAUDHARY et al. 1990; SIEGALL et al. 1990). For DT, it has meant the use of CRM107, with mutations at residues 390 and 525 in the binding domain (GREENFIELD et al. 1987). And for ricin it has meant the inactivation of the B chain by the use of glycopeptides (LAMBERT et al. 1991) or mutations in sugar-binding motifs that reduce cell surface binding (FRANKEL et al. 1996, 1997).

3 Intracellular Processing – Cleavage and Reduction

Each toxin has a proteolytic cleavage site and a key disulfide bond that holds the molecule together even after cleavage. This means that release of the catalytic domain requires proteolysis followed by reduction. Since full-length molecules do not translocate to the cytosol, toxicity is dependent on the timely processing (i.e., cleavage and reduction) of the native toxin.

Of the type 2 RIPs, ricin has been studied most extensively. When isolated from the castor plant, ricin is a heterodimer consisting of a 32,000 dalton A chain (RTA) and a 32,000 dalton B chain (RTB). Ricin is synthesized as a proenzyme with a leader peptide upstream of the A chain and a 12 residue linking peptide which joins the A and B chains; both are removed by proteolytic processing in the plant to form the mature ricin heterodimer (HARLEY and LORD 1985). The A and B chains are held together by noncovalent forces, but are also secured by a disulfide bond between Cys-259 of RTA and Cys-4 of RTB, which assures toxin integrity even at very low concentrations (LEWIS and YOULE 1986). After binding and entry into mammalian cells, the A-B heterodimer of ricin must be reduced to allow the A chain to translocate to the cytosol. While the reduction step remains a simple concept, there are no data to indicate either the intracellular location or the mechanism of reduction.

DT is secreted from its host as a single chain protein. It's arginine rich loop at the COOH-terminal portion of the enzymatic domain is susceptible to cleavage in both bacterial and mammalian cell culture media. Because of this, DT is often found as a nicked protein held together by the disulfide bond joining cysteines 186 and 201. The cleavage of intact toxin by mammalian cells is likely to involve the action of a serine protease such as furin or urokinase (CHIRON et al. 1994; WILLIAMS et al. 1990). The reduction of nicked DT by mammalian cells has been studied by RYSER et al. (1991; MANDEL et al. 1993). They reported that nicked DT can be cleaved at the plasma membrane by thiol exchange and may involve the action of protein disulfide isomerase.

At neutral pH, PE is relative resistant to protease attack. However, within the acidic environment of the endosome PE changes conformation and is rendered sensitive to furin mediated cleavage (CHIRON et al. 1994). Cleavage by furin is dependent on the presence of P1 and P4 arginines at residues 279 and 276, respectively. Cells that lack furin are PE resistant. Transfection of a cDNA encoding wild-type furin restores toxin sensitivity (MOEHRING et al. 1993) to cells lacking functional furin. After cleavage, PE is reduced to fragments of 28 and 37kDa (OGATA et al. 1990). To date this latter step in the toxin pathway has not been well characterized.

3.1 Cytosolic Activity

Once RTA has been translocated to the cytoplasm, it attacks the large subunit of ribosomes. RTA is an N-glycosidase enzyme, removing a specific adenine base from a very conservative region of the 28S rRNA (ENDO et al. 1987). The susceptible adenine base lies in a context GAGA, part of the loop of a vital stem-loop substructure of the ribosome. Its removal prevents the ribosome from interacting properly with elongation factors required for protein synthesis. RTA has a

Km = 0.1 (M for rabbit reticulocyte ribosomes) and a $k$cat = 1500min (OLSNES et al. 1975). These numbers show that the toxin has evolved to near perfection; its catalytic action is diffusion limited and no better enzyme is theoretically possible for this reaction.

The translocation of an active fragment to the cytosol can only cause cell death if the enzymatic portion of the toxin survives the degradative capacity of the proteasome system and other cytosolic proteases. Properties that render toxin fragments resistant to destruction have not been described.

4 Immunotoxin Design and Testing

Recombinant immunotoxins are generated by deleting the DNA encoding the binding portion of toxins and replacing it with antibody sequences (MURPHY and VANDERSPEK 1995; PASTAN et al. 1995). This strategy has been reported most often for the bacterial toxins PE and DT, with the generation of plant recombinant immunotoxins lagging behind. However, recent studies have shown that mutated B chains (FRANKEL et al. 1997) or selected A chains e.g. Bryodin (SIEGALL et al., in press) can be fused with cell binding ligands or antibodies to generate active immunotoxins.

Because recombinant immunotoxins are made by gene fusion technology, certain constraints are inherent in their construction. A ligand fused with domains II and III of PE has to be placed at the NH_2-terminal of the construction. This means that the COOH-terminal of the ligand is joined via a peptide bond with the NH_2-terminal of domain II. If the ligand requires a free COOH-terminal to mediate receptor binding, this kind of construction is likely to exhibit diminished binding activity. The same situation but with an opposite orientation applies to immunotoxins made with DT.

Single chain antibodies are composed of the variable light and variable heavy chains of a monoclonal antibody (Fig. 3). Routinely, to hold these two chains together, a 15 amino acid flexible peptide linker is used to tether the COOH-terminal of one chain with the NH_2-terminal of the second chain (BIRD et al. 1988; HUSTON et al. 1988). While this approach facilitates expression of the recombinant antibody from a single transcript, the product is not always stable. Unstable single chain antibodies can be stabilized by the introduction of novel disulfide bonds into the framework segments of the variable chains (REITER et al. 1994a,b). Residues that are opposed and separated by the appropriate distance are modified to create novel cysteine residues, one each in the light and heavy chains. The light chain with a free sulfhydryl can then be linked by a disulfide bond with a heavy chain construct to form a disulfide stabilized Fv (fragment variable) immunotoxin. Such an approach has been used successfully to generate several very stable recombinant immunotoxins.

Immunotoxin expresssion in E. coli

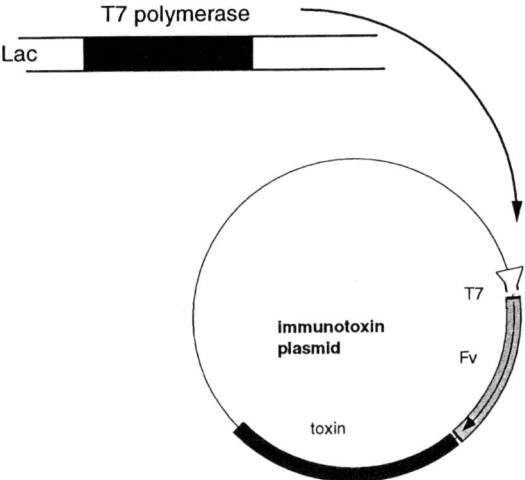

Fig. 2. Recombinant immunotoxin expression

Recombinant immunotoxin genes are often cloned in an expression plasmid downstream of the T7 promoter (Fig. 2). Plasmids are transformed into an expression host, typically *E. coli* strain BL21(λDE3), developed by STUDIER and MOFFATT (1986). The strain produces T7 polymerase in response to induction of the lactose operon. Immunotoxins are usually produced within the *E. coli* cell and are later recovered from inclusion bodies by denaturation and renaturation. The renatured material is then typically purified by Q Sepharose, Mono Q and HPLC size exclusion chromatography (BUCHNER et al. 1992). The synthesis and release of immunotoxins from mammalian cells was reported recently (CHEN et al. 1997). This kind of production may have certain advantages for the local killing of tumor cells especially if transfected T cells can be engineered to secrete the immunotoxin (CHEN et al. 1997).

Purified immunotoxins are tested for cytotoxicity in the range of 0.1–100ng/ml. After an overnight incubation on both target and nontarget cells, the level of new protein synthesis is determined. Immunotoxins that exhibit IC_{50} values below 10ng/ml for target cells and above 1000ng/ml for nontarget cells are considered potent and selective enough for testing in tumor models. Mice are injected with the appropriate tumor xenograft. After several days to allow the tumor to get established, immunotoxin treatments are given (immunotoxin injections on days 5, 7 and 9 are typical). Anti-tumor activity and toxicity to mice are assessed. A therapeutic window is established whereby the therapeutic dose is compared with the toxic dose (the LD_{50} is divided by the dose giving complete regressions of tumor).

Recombinant Fv immunotoxins

Fig. 3. Fv antibody-toxin constructs – single chain and disulfide stabilized

scFv immunotoxin

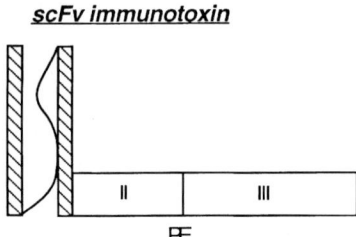

dsFv immunotoxin

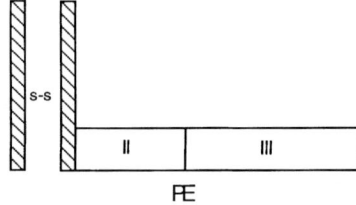

scFv = single chain Fv

dsFv = disulfide stabilized Fv

5 Conclusion

It is possible to design and produce wholly recombinant immunotoxins, comprised of truncated toxin molecules joined with tumor-targeting agents that exhibit cytotoxic activity for target cell lines and anti-tumor activity in model systems. Results of ongoing clinical trials will determine the utility of these agents.

References

Allured VS, Collier RJ, Carroll SF, McKay DB (1986) Structure of exotoxin A of Pseudomonas aeruginosa at 30 Angstrom. Proc Natl Acad Sci USA 83:1320–1324

Baenziger JU, Fiete D (1979) Structural determinants of Ricinus communis agglutinin and toxin specificity for oligosaccharides. J Biol Chem 254:9795–9799

Bennett MJ, Eisenberg D (1994) Refined structure of monomeric diphtheria toxin at 23 A resolution. Protein Sci 3:1464–1475
Bird RE, Hardman KD, Jacobson JW, Johnson S, Kaufman BM, Lee SM, Lee T, Pope SH, Riordan GS, Whitlow M (1988) Single-chain antigen-binding proteins [published erratum appears in Science 1989 Apr 28;244(4903):409]. Science 242:423–426
Buchner J, Pastan I, Brinkmann U (1992) A method for increasing the yield of properly folded recombinant fusion proteins: single-chain immunotoxins from renaturation of bacterial inclusion bodies. Anal Biochem 205:263–270
Cavallaro U, Soria MR (1995) Targeting plant toxins to the urokinase and alpha 2-macroglobulin receptors. Semin Cancer Biol 6:269–278
Cavallaro U, Nykjaer A, Nielsen M, Soria MR (1995) Alpha 2-macroglobulin receptor mediates binding and cytotoxicity of plant ribosome-inactivating proteins. Eur J Biochem 232:165–171
Chaudhary VK, Jinno Y, FitzGerald D, Pastan I (1990a) Pseudomonas exotoxin contains a specific sequence at the carboxyl terminus that is required for cytotoxicity. Proc Natl Acad Sci USA 87:308–312
Chaudhary VK, Jinno Y, Gallo MG, FitzGerald D, Pastan I (1990b) Mutagenesis of Pseudomonas exotoxin in identification of sequences responsible for the animal toxicity. J Biol Chem 265:16306–16310
Chen SY, Yang AG, Chen JD, Kute T, King CR, Collier J, Cong Y, Yao C, Huang XF (1997) Potent antitumour activity of a new class of tumour-specific killer cells. Nature 385:78–80
Chiron MF, Fryling CM, FitzGerald DJ (1994) Cleavage of pseudomonas exotoxin and diphtheria toxin by a furin-like protease prepared from beef liver. J Biol Chem 269:18167–18176
Choe S, Bennett MJ, Fujii G, Kantardjieff KA, Collier RJ, Eisenberg D (1992) The crystal structure of diphtheria toxin. Nature 357:216–222
Collier RJ (1988) Structure-activity relationships in diphtheria toxin and Pseudomonas aeruginosa exotoxin A. Cancer Treat Res 37:25–35
Endo Y, Mitsui K, Motizuki M, Tsurugi K (1987) Mechanism of action of ricin and related toxic lectins on eukaryotic ribosomes: the site and characteristics of the modification in 28S rRNA caused by the toxins. J Biol Chem 262:5908–5912
FitzGerald DJ, Fryling CM, Zdanovsky A, Saelinger CB, Kounnas M, Winkles JA, Strickland D, Leppla S (1995) Pseudomonas exotoxin-mediated selection yields cells with altered expression of low-density lipoprotein receptor-related protein [published erratum appears in J Cell Biol 1995 Aug;130(4):1015]. J Cell Biol 129:1533–1541
Frankel AE, Burbage C, Fu T, Tagge E, Chandler J, Willingham MC (1996) Ricin toxin contains at least three galactose-binding sites located in B chain subdomains 1 alpha, 1 beta, and 2 gamma. Biochemistry 35:14749–14756
Frankel AE, Fu T, Burbage C, Chandler J, Willingham MC, Tagge EP (1997) IL2 fused to lectin-deficient ricin is toxic to human leukemia cells expressing the IL2 receptor. Leukemia 11:22–30
Gray GL, Smith DH, Baldridge JS, Harkins RN, Vasil ML, Chen EY, Heyneker HL (1984) Cloning, nucleotide sequence, and expression in E. coli of the exotoxin a structural gene of Pseudomonas aeruginosa. Proc Natl Acad Sci USA 81:2645–2649
Greenfield L, Bjorn MJ, Horn G, Fong D, Buck GA, Collier RJ, Kaplan DA (1983) Nucleotide sequence of the structural gene for diphtheria toxin carried by corynebacteriophage beta. Proc Natl Acad Sci USA 80:6853–6857
Greenfield L, Johnson VG, Youle RJ (1987) Mutations in diphtheria toxin separate binding from entry and amplify immunotoxin selectivity. Science 238:536–539
Harley SM, Lord JM (1985) In vitro endoproteolytic cleavage of castor bean lectin precursors. Plant Sci 41:111–116
Huston JS, Levinson D, Mudgett HM, Tai MS, Novotny J, Margolies MN, Ridge RJ, Bruccoleri RE, Haber E, Crea R et al (1988) Protein engineering of antibody binding sites: recovery of specific activity in an anti-digoxin single-chain Fv analogue produced in Escherichia coli. Proc Natl Acad Sci USA 85:5879–5883
Katzin BJ, Collins EJ, Robertus JD (1991) Structure of ricin A-chain at 25A resolution. Prot Struct Funct Genet 10:251–259
Kaul P, Silverman J, Shen WH, Blanke SR, Huynh PD, Finkelstein A, Collier RJ (1996) Roles of Glu 349 and Asp 352 in membrane insertion and translocation by diphtheria toxin. Prot Sci 5:687–92
Kounnas MZ, Morris RE, Thompson MR, FitzGerald DJ, Strickland DK, Saelinger CB (1992) The alpha 2-macroglobulin receptor/low density lipoprotein receptor-related protein binds and internalizes pseudomonas exotoxin A. J Biol Chem 267:12420–12423

Lamb FI, Roberts LM, Lord JM (1985) Nucleotide sequence of cloned cDNA coding for preproricin. Eur J Biochem 148:265–270

Lambert JM, McIntyre G, Gauthier N, Zullo D, Rao V, Steeves RM, Goldmacher VS, Blattler WA (1991) The galactose-binding sites of the cytotoxic lectin ricin can be chemically blocked in high yields with reactive ligands prepared by chemical modification of glycopeptides containing triantennary N-linked oligosaccharides. Biochemistry 30:3234–3247

Lemichez E, Bomsel M, Devilliers G, vanderSpek J, Murphy JR, Lukianov EV, Olsnes S, Boquet P (1997) Membrane translocation of diphtheria toxin fragment A exploits early to late endosome trafficking machinery. Mol Microbiol 23:445–457

Lewis MS, Youle RJ (1986) Ricin subunit association Thermodynamics and the role of the disulfide bond in toxicity. J Biol Chem 261:11571–11577

Li M, Dyda F, Benhar I, Pastan I, Davies DR (1995) The crystal structure of Pseudomonas aeruginosa exotoxin domain III with nicotinamide and AMP: conformational differences with the intact exotoxin. Proc Natl Acad Sci USA 92:9308–9312

Li M, Dyda F, Benhar I, Pastan I, Davies DR (1996) Crystal structure of the catalytic domain of Pseudomonas exotoxin A complexed with a nicotinamide adenine dinucleotide analog: implications for the activation process and for ADP ribosylation. Proc Natl Acad Sci USA 93:6902–6906

Mandel R, Ryser HJ, Ghani F, Wu M, Peak D (1993) Inhibition of a reductive function of the plasma membrane by bacitracin and antibodies against protein disulfide-isomerase. Proc Natl Acad Sci USA 90:4112–4116

Moehring JM, Inocencio NM, Robertson BJ, Moehring TJ (1993) Expression of mouse furin in a Chinese hamster cell resistant to Pseudomonas exotoxin A and viruses complements the genetic lesion. J Biol Chem 268:2590–2594

Montfort W, Villafranca JE, Monzingo AF, Ernst SR, Katzin B, Rutenber E, Xuong NH, Hamlin R, Robertus JD (1987) The three-dimensional structure of ricin at 28A. J Biol Chem 262:5398–5403

Murphy JR, vanderSpek JC (1995) Targeting diphtheria toxin to growth factor receptors. Semin Cancer Biol 6:259–267

Naglich JG, Metherall JE, Russell DW, Eidels L (1992a) Expression cloning of a diphtheria toxin receptor: identity with a heparin-binding EGF-like growth factor precursor. Cell 69:1051–1061

Naglich JG, Rolf JM, Eidels L (1992b) Expression of functional diphtheria toxin receptors on highly toxin-sensitive mouse cells that specifically bind radioiodinated toxin. Proc Natl Acad Sci USA 89:2170–2174

Ogata M, Chaudhary VK, Pastan I, FitzGerald DJ (1990) Processing of Pseudomonas exotoxin by a cellular protease results in the generation of a 37,000-Da toxin fragment that is translocated to the cytosol. J Biol Chem 265:20678–20685

Olsnes S, Fernandez-Puentes C, Carrasco L, Vazquez D (1975) Ribosome inactivation by the toxic lectins abrin and ricin Kinetics of the enzymatic activity of the toxin A-chains. Eur J Biochem 60:281–288

Pastan IH, Pai LH, Brinkmann U, Fitzgerald DJ (1995) Recombinant toxins: new therapeutic agents for cancer. Ann NY Acad Sci 758:345–354

Pelham HRB, Roberts LM, Lord JM (1992) Toxin entry: how reversible is the secretory pathway? Trends Cell Biol 2:183–185

Reiter Y, Brinkmann U, Kreitman RJ, Jung SH, Lee B, Pastan I (1994a) Stabilization of the Fv fragments in recombinant immunotoxins by disulfide bonds engineered into conserved framework regions. Biochemistry 33:5451–5459

Reiter Y, Brinkmann U, Webber KO, Jung SH, Lee B, Pastan I (1994b) Engineering interchain disulfide bonds into conserved framework regions of Fv fragments: improved biochemical characteristics of recombinant immunotoxins containing disulfide-stabilized Fv. Protein Eng 7:697–704

Rutenber E, Robertus JD (1991) Structure of ricin B-chain at 25A resolution. Prot Struct Funct Genet 10:260–269

Ryser HJ, Mandel R, Ghani F (1991) Cell surface sulfhydryls are required for the cytotoxicity of diphtheria toxin but not of ricin in Chinese hamster ovary cells. J Biol Chem 266:18439–18442

Sandvig K, Ryd M, Garred O, Schweda E, Holm PK, van Deurs B (1994) Retrograde transport from the Golgi complex to the ER of both Shiga toxin and the nontoxic Shiga B-fragment is regulated by butyric acid and cAMP. J Cell Biol 126:53–64

Siegall CB, FitzGerald DJ, Pastan I (1990) Cytotoxicity of IL6-PE40 and derivatives on tumor cells expressing a range of interleukin 6 receptor levels. J Biol Chem 265:16318–16323

Studier FW, Moffatt BA (1986) Use of bacteriophage T7 polymerase to direct selective expression of cloned gene. J Mol Biol 189:113–130

Wales R, Roberts LM, Lord JM (1993) Addition of an endoplasmic reticulum retrieval sequence to ricin A chain significantly increases its cytotoxicity to mammalian cells. J Biol Chem 268:23986–23990

Weiss MS, Blanke SR, Collier RJ, Eisenberg D (1995) Structure of the isolated catalytic domain of diphtheria toxin. Biochemistry 34:773–781

Williams DP, Wen Z, Watson RS, Boyd J, Strom TB, Murphy JR (1990) Cellular processing of the interleukin-2 fusion toxin DAB486-IL-2 and efficient delivery of diphtheria fragment A to the cytosol of target cells requires Arg194. J Biol Chem 265:20673–20677

Zentz C, Frenoy JP, Bourrillon R (1978) Binding of galactose and lactose to ricin Equilibrium studies. Biochim Biophys Acta 536:18–26

The Emerging Role of Ricin A-Chain Immunotoxins in Leukemia and Lymphoma

A. ENGERT,[1] E.A. SAUSVILLE,[2] and E. VITETTA[3]

1 Introduction	13
2 Preclinical Studies with Ricin A-Chain Immunotoxins	14
2.1 First Generation Ricin A-Chain Immunotoxins	14
2.2 Second Generation Immunotoxins	15
2.3 Recombinant Ricin A-Chain Immunotoxins	16
2.4 Cytotoxic Properties of Ricin A-Chain Immunotoxin In Vitro	17
2.5 Tissue Distribution and Toxicology of Ricin A-Chain Immunotoxins in Rodents	18
2.6 The Performance of Immunotoxins in Animals	18
2.7 Immunotoxin Cocktails	20
3 Clinical Trials with Ricin A-Chain Immunotoxins	20
3.1 Anti-CD5-Ricin A-Chain	20
3.2 Anti-breast Cancer Immunotoxin 260F9-rRTA	21
3.3 Anti-B Cell Immunotoxins RFB4-dgRTA and HD 37-dgRTA	21
3.4 Anti-CD25-dgRTA	24
3.5 Vascular Leak Syndrome	24
3.6 Human Anti-immunotoxin Antibodies	25
4 Perspectives	25
4.1 New Immunotoxins	25
4.2 Vascular Targeting	26
4.3 Treatment of Minimal Residual Disease	27
5 Summary	27
References	28

1 Introduction

Although some malignancies can be cured by conventional modalities including surgery, radiotherapy and polychemotherapy, many cancer patients still ultimately die of their disease. The major reason for this poor outcome is the persistence or selection of cells which are refractory to conventional treatment. These cells might

---

[1] Department I for Internal Medicine, University of Cologne, 50924 Cologne, Germany, e-mail: a.engert@uni-koeln.de
[2] Developmental Therapeutics Program, National Cancer Institute, Bethesda, MD 20892, USA
[3] Cancer Immunobiology Center and Department of Microbiology, The University of Texas, Southwestern Medical Center, Dallas, TX 75235, USA

be eradicated by new immunotherapeutic agents with different modes of action. In this regard, monoclonal antibodies (Moabs) have become available in limitless quantities making more selective immunotherapy feasible. These Moabs can bind to well-defined antigens expressed on the surface of malignant cells. Unfortunately, many Moabs have very weak or no anti-tumor activity when used in their native form. Thus, Moabs are often linked to radioisotopes or toxins to increase their toxicity. Immunotoxins (ITs) are constructed by chemically or genetically linking the antibody moiety to a potent bacterial or plant toxin. To date, the most widely used toxin is ricin, which is derived from the seeds of *Ricinus communis* (castor bean).

In this chapter, we describe the preparation of ricin A-chain (RTA)-containing ITs and summarize recent data on their preclinical and clinical use.

2 Preclinical Studies with Ricin A-Chain Immunotoxins

2.1 First Generation Ricin A-Chain Immunotoxins

To prepare effective ITs for in vivo therapy, the ligand and toxin must be coupled in such a way as to remain stable in both the bloodstream and the tissues and yet be labile within the target cell so that the toxic portion can be released into the cytosol. RTA-containing ITs have been prepared almost exclusively by chemical cross-linking because it is difficult to genetically engineer an IT with a disulfide bond between the antibody and the toxin (O'HARE et al. 1990; SPOONER et al. 1994).

Linkers used to couple ligands to RTA must introduce a disulfide bond between the ligand and the RTA. Table 1 summarizes the linkers that have been used to accomplish this. Bonds that cannot be reduced (e.g., thioether bonds) render these ITs either much less toxic or nontoxic (MASUHO et al. 1982), suggesting that the RTA is released from the ligand by intracellular reduction. The linker used to couple the RTA to the ligand is usually a heterobifunctional cross-linker which introduces an activated thiol group into the ligand. When the derivatized ligand is mixed with the reduced RTA, the free thiol group in the RTA (its former site of attachment to the RTB) displaces the leaving group from the activated thiol group introduced into the ligand and forms the disulfide linkage. Since only one or two activated thiol groups are usually introduced into the ligand (WAWRZYNCZAK and THORPE 1987a; GROS et al. 1985), the resultant IT is contaminated with both free RTA and free ligand. The free RTA, much of the unreacted antibody, and high molecular weight aggregates are removed by gel permeation chromatography (CUMBER et al. 1985). The remaining free antibody is removed by adsorbing the IT by its RTA moiety to columns of either blue Sepharose (KNOWLES and THORPE 1987) or immobilized anti-RTA antibodies (VITETTA et al. 1987), washing away the free antibody and eluting the RTA-containing IT (IT-A) with high salt or low pH. It should be noted that while contamination with RTA is not usually a

Table 1. Linkers used to prepare ricin A-chain-containing immunotoxins

Cross-Linker[+]	IT Structure
None	Fab–SS–Ⓐ
SATA	IgG–NH–CO–CH$_2$–SS–Ⓐ
SPDP	IgG–NH–CO–CH$_2$–CH$_2$–SS–Ⓐ
2-IT	IgG–NH–C(=NH$_2^+$)–CH$_2$–CH$_2$–CH–SS–Ⓐ
SMPT	IgG–NH–CO–⬡–CH(CH$_3$)–SS–Ⓐ

*From Wawrzynczak and Thorpe (Wawrzynczak and Thorpe 1987).
[+] 2-IT = 2-iminothiolane; SATA = N-succinimidyl-S-thioacetate; SPDP, N-succinimidyl-3-(2-pyridyldihio) propionate;
SMPT = N-succinimidyl-oxycarbonyl-a-methyl-a(2-pyrodyldithio) tuluene.

problem in vivo, contamination with free antibody can present a significant problem (BLAKEY and THORPE 1988), since the half-life of an intact antibody is much longer than that of an IT (BLAKEY et al. 1987; BOURRIE et al. 1986; BYERS et al. 1987). Thus, after a period of time in vivo, the free antibody is present in the blood and tissues in greater amounts than the IT and can compete for binding sites on the target cells, effectively reducing the potency of the IT.

2.2 Second Generation Immunotoxins

The "first generation" heterobifunctional cross-linkers, such as SPDP or 2-IT, generated disulfide bonds that were quite unstable in vivo, releasing RTA and antibody with a $T_{1/2}$ of 6–8h (FULTON et al. 1988a; BLAKEY et al. 1987; THORPE et al. 1987a). Breakdown was probably due to reduction by glutathione, albumin, and other thiol-containing molecules in the bloodstream and tissues. This problem has been solved by the synthesis of new cross-linkers, e.g., SMPT (THORPE et al. 1987b), which introduce hindered disulfide bonds having phenyl and/or methyl groups onto carbon atoms adjacent to the disulfide bond. ITs prepared with these hindered cross-linkers are much more stable ($T_{1/2}$, approximately 2 days) (THORPE et al. 1987b) and have improved anti-tumor activity (THORPE et al. 1988) compared to their predecessors.

In addition to utilizing better cross-linkers, some second generation ITs were also smaller. Since Fab and some Fab' fragments of antibodies have a free cysteine residue near the hinge region (STANWORTH and TURNER 1978), these can be used to form a disulfide bridge with the free cysteine residue of the RTA. The coupling is generally accomplished by activating the thiol group in the Fab/Fab' fragment with Ellman's reagent (to provide a good leaving group) and mixing the derivatized Fab/

Fab' with the reduced RTA (RASO and GRIFFIN 1980). The Fab/Fab'-RTA then forms by a thiol-disulfide exchange reaction. Since the thiol group of the Fab/Fab' fragment is distant from its antigen-combining site (STANWORTH and TURNER 1978), and since there is usually only one free thiol group on the fragments derived from most subclasses of murine Moabs (PARHAM 1983; SVASTI and MILSTEIN 1972), this assures the attachment of one RTA per Fab/Fab' fragment at a site distant from the combining site. Unlike the IgG-RTA, such constructs, therefore, retain full antigen-binding activity.

RTA is glycosylated and contains mannose and fucose-terminating oligosaccharides (KIMURA et al. 1988). These sugars are recognized by avid receptors on both the parenchymal and nonparenchymal cells of the liver and by cells of the reticuloendothelial system (RES) (BLAKEY et al. 1988; SKILLETER et al. 1981). Hence, IT-RTAs prepared from native RTA are cleared rapidly from the bloodstream, and this may have been at least partially responsible for the failure of first generation IT-RTAs to reach their target cells in vivo and elicit their intended antitumor effects. In addition, entrapment of the IT-RTAs by the liver results in liver damage (JANSEN et al. 1982), although this is fairly modest because IT-RTAs taken up through the carbohydrate recognition pathways are probably routed to the lysosomes and destroyed.

The problem of liver recognition of RTA was solved by destroying, i.e., "deglycosylating" the mannose and fucose residues on the ricin molecule by a simple procedure involving periodate oxidation and cyanoborohydride reduction at low pH (THORPE et al. 1985b). This procedure does not affect the enzymatic activity of RTA or its ability to function as an IT (BLAKEY et al. 1987). ITs constructed with deglycosylated RTA (dgRTA) prepared with intact antibodies and stable linkers are long-lived in mice lacking target cells for which the IT is specific. The IT is cleared only about twice as quickly as is native mouse IgG (THORPE et al. 1987a, THORPE et al. 1988).

2.3 Recombinant Ricin A-Chain Immunotoxins

The cDNA encoding the precursor of ricin (preproricin) has been cloned (LAMB et al. 1985) and the segment of DNA encoding the A-chain has been expressed in *Escherichia coli* (O'HARE et al. 1987). The expressed RTA was devoid of carbohydrate and did not localize in the liver. A technique was also developed for synthesizing cytotoxic RTA fusion proteins in *E. coli* (O'HARE et al. 1990). The gene for the ligand (staphylococcal protein-A) was ligated to the DNA encoding RTA via an intervening spacer sequence derived from the diphtheria toxin gene. The single chain fusion protein was expressed in *E. coli*. The function of the diphtheria toxin spacer was to form a disulfide-bonded loop between the ligand and the A-chain which could be subsequently nicked with trypsin to yield a two chain structure in which the ligand and the A-chain were joined by a disulfide bond. The nicked fusion protein was highly cytotoxic to Ig-coated target cells in vitro. An active IT prepared with an anti-breast cancer Moab biochemically cross-linked to recombinant RTA has been prepared and tested in humans (BJORN et al. 1985; FRANKEL et al. 1985; GOULD et al. 1989).

2.4 Cytotoxic Properties of Ricin A-Chain Immunotoxin In Vitro

RTA-containing ITs show virtually complete specificity in their cytotoxic effect on target cells in vitro because their only means of binding to cells is through the ligand portion of the IT. Fc binding, if it occurs, appears not to route the IT to an intracellular compartment favorable for RTA release and cell killing. The major disadvantage of IT-RTAs, however, is that they have variable cytotoxic potencies (BJORN et al. 1985); only about 25% of such ITs are potently toxic to their target cells.

It is now generally accepted that a variety of factors concerning Moabs or ligands play major roles in determining whether or not they will make effective ITs (GHETIE et al. 1988; RAMAKRISHNAN and HOUSTON 1984a; SHEN et al. 1988; ENGERT et al. 1990a). These variables include specificity, affinity, internalization and intracellular routing. For example, those antibodies or ligands with low binding affinity generally make poor ITs while those with high affinity are usually quite good. This is probably the main reason why Fab'-RTAs having only one antigen-combining site tend to be threefold to several 100-fold less effective than their intact antibody counterparts, which have higher avidity because of their bivalency. Secondly, the cell surface molecule that the antibody recognizes plays a key role in determining the efficacy of the IT (PRESS et al. 1986, 1988; MAY et al. 1990). In general, cell surface molecules such as growth factor receptors, which continuously recycle into endosomal compartments or which can be induced to do so by binding to an antibody or other ligand, make effective targets for ITs. Cell surface molecules which are not readily internalized or which are internalized into intracellular compartments unfavorable for RTA translocation (e.g., the lysosomes) make poor ITs no matter how high their avidity. It has also been reported that the target antigen, which is often a large cell surface glycoprotein, can have numerous epitopes and that antibodies against different epitopes can differ in their effectiveness as ITs (PRESS et al. 1988; MAY et al. 1990). The most likely explanation for this finding is that Moabs may have to recognize epitopes close to the plasma membrane for the RTA to insert into the membrane and be translocated across the membrane into the cytosol after endocytosis.

RTA-containing ITs that are weakly effective often show greatly improved toxicity in the presence of lysosomotropic amines (e.g., ammonium chloride, chloroquine) (CASELLAS et al. 1984; RAMAKRISHNAN and HOUSTON 1984), carboxylic ionophores (e.g., monensin) (RASO and LAWRENCE 1984), RTB chains (McINTOSH et al. 1983; YOULE and NEVILLE 1982) and Moab-RTB chains (VITETTA et al. 1983, 1984). Two- to 1,000-fold improvements in IT potency are common. The lysosomotropic amines and the carboxylic ionophores probably work by slowing the fusion of endosomes with lysosomes (RASO 1988) (where RTA-chains are enzymatically destroyed) or by delaying the transit of the IT through a compartment favorable for RTA translocation, for example, the transGolgi. The RTB chains and Moab-RTB chains probably work by protecting the RTA from degradation or enhancing their translocation across the membranes of intracellular compartments. Lysosomotropic amines also potentiate the nonspecific activity of any contaminating toxin or RTB (FULTON et al. 1986). Exquisite care must, therefore, be taken to eliminate RTB or toxin from a purified IT or enhancement may result from contamination rather than from a direct effect on the IT.

An assay has been developed to screen Moabs in order to predict which ones will make effective ITs (TILL et al. 1988). This assay involves binding the Moab (in the form of a tissue culture supernatant, ascites, or purified antibody) to the target cells and then treating the coated cells with a secondary Fab' or Fab fragment of an anti-mouse, rat, or human immunoglobulin linked to an RTA (TILL et al. 1988). In most cases, the degree of killing predicts quite accurately the potency of that Moab when it is coupled directly to the RTA-chain. This assay is an important development since previously each Moab had to undergo time-consuming purification, linkage to the RTA-chain, and evaluation by cytotoxicity assays on target cells.

2.5 Tissue Distribution and Toxicology of Ricin A-Chain Immunotoxins in Rodents

Of all the ITs so far studied in depth, only those prepared with dgRTA appear not to cause liver damage in rodents. At doses of IT-dgRTAs approaching the LD_{50}, the only normal tissue damage visible in mice and primates is in the crypts of Lieberkuhn, the small intestine (JANSEN et al. 1982), the proximal tubule of the kidney (JANSEN et al. 1982), and skeletal muscle (FULTON et al. 1988). In vitro, dgRTA/RTA can damage human endothelial cells (SOLER-RODRIGUEZ et al. 1993). None of these effects appear to be severe enough to account for death, and the cause of death at high doses of IT-As is currently known. The Fab'-dgRTAs induce similar toxic side effects except that, in some experiments, the myositis is more marked, possibly because Fab'-dgRTAs permeate extravascular tissues more readily because of their smaller size. By contrast, the LD_{50} of Fab'-dgRTAs is three- to fivefold greater (on a total protein basis) than that of IgG-dgRTAs (FULTON et al. 1988), probably because they are more rapidly cleared (FULTON et al. 1988).

2.6 The Performance of Immunotoxins in Animals

Animal models have facilitated the evaluation and refinement of different types of IT constructs. First-generation IT-As containing native RTA and unstable linkers were developed into second-generation IT-As. These contain dgRTA and stable linkers and have dramatically superior anti-tumor activity as compared with their predecessors (VITETTA et al. 1987; THORPE et al. 1988). Moreover, Fab'-dgRTAs have been compared with IgG-dgRTAs and, depending on the test system, have shown weaker or equivalent anti-tumor activity, but lower immunogenicity (FULTON et al. 1988).

Table 2. Curative effect of different immunotoxins in SCID mice with disseminated human tumors

Human xenograft	Tumor type	Inoculation	Immunotoxin construct	Treatment Specificity	Time after tumor inoculation	Therapeutic[a] effect (%CR)
L540Cy	Hodgkin's lymphoma	i.v.	RFT5-dg RTA	CD25	1 day	95
			IRac-dg RTA	70KD	12 days	46
					1 day	93
Daudi	Burkitt's lymphoma	i.v.	RFB4-dgRTA + HD37(Fab)$_2$	CD22/ CD19	1 day	100
Daudi	Burkitt's lymphoma	i.v.	RFB4-dgRTA + HD37-dgRTA + Doxorubicin (cytoxan) (campothecin)	CD22/ CD19	1 day	100

[a] Percent of mice in complete remission; CR: longterm, tumor-free survival

It has been established in animal models that marked anti-tumor effects, prolonged remissions, and even cures (THORPE et al. 1985a, 1988; JANSEN et al. 1980) can be achieved with doses of RTA-ITs that are well tolerated (Table 2). In general, tumors that are readily accessible to the bloodstream appear to be most responsive. In addition, the effectiveness of combinatorial therapy has been well documented in animal models (GHETIE et al. 1996). For example, access of ITs to solid tumors and anti-tumor activity can be improved by coadministration of adrenergic blockers, which may act by selectively constricting normal vasculature and increasing the tumor-to-normal-tissue perfusion ratio (SMYTH et al. 1987). Coadministration of the carboxylic ionophore monensin, either free (RAMAKRISHNAN et al. 1989) or conjugated to serum albumin (CASELLAS and JANSEN 1988), can also potentiate the anti-tumor activity of an IT-A. It will probably be necessary to give ITs in combination with conventional chemotherapeutic drugs or radiotherapy because the modes of action of the different therapies do not overlap; thus, the resistant mutants that escape one type of therapy succumb to the other. In this regard, results in SCID mice xenografted with human tumors demonstrate that ITs work well in combination with chemotherapy (GHETIE et al. 1994, 1996).

The administration of ITs to animals with intact immune systems leads to an antibody response against both components, precluding repeated treatments. Immunosuppressive regimens can delay anti-IT responses, but may also compromise the host's ability to suppress the growth of residual tumor. One way to decrease the immunogenicity of ITs is to modify them with monomethoxy-polyethyleneglycol (PEG). PEG has been used to decrease the immunogenicity and increase the blood residence time of various enzymes (KATRE 1993) and Igs (KITAMURA et al. 1991, 1996). PEG-RTA has been conjugated to an anti-breast cancer antibody but the resulting IT showed a tenfold decrease in its ability to inhibit protein synthesis in a cell-free system. Unexpectedly, its cytotoxicity in vitro against a breast cancer cell line was unaffected. Because RTA has only two lysine residues (susceptible to derivatization with PEG), the number of PEG molecules per RTA may not be sufficient to confer a longer half-life and lower immunogenicity (V. GHETIE, unpublished results).

More recent studies involve novel immunosuppressives agents which block either T/B cell stimulation or costimulation (LAMAN et al. 1996; LENSCHOW et al. 1996; SIEGALL et al. 1997) and preliminary results are encouraging (E. NOON and E. S. VITETTA, submitted to Clin, Cancer Res. The effect of immunosuppresive agents on the immunogenicity and efficacy of an Immunotoxin in mice). However, until specific tolerance to an IT can be induced, it is probably advisable to administer the IT in a short course prior to the development of a primary antibody response.

2.7 Immunotoxin Cocktails

Another problem in using Moab-based anti-tumor reagents is the selection of antigen-deficient mutants causing late relapses in experimental animals (THORPE et al. 1988). A solution would be to use IT cocktails, i.e., combinations of ITs directed against different antigens or epitopes on the same target cell. Superior effects of IT cocktails have been demonstrated for both, non-Hodgkin's and Hodgkin's lymphoma (NHL) (GHETIE et al. 1992; ENGERT et al. 1995). Lymphomas are well suited for the use of IT cocktails since several potent ITs against different target antigens are available. The superiority of the IT cocktails can be explained by the fact that most tumors contain a proportion of cells which express the target antigen at low density at the time of treatment. These cells might be a "dormant" subpopulation having reduced numbers of activation markers which are nevertheless capable of fully reentering proliferation (PANTEL et al. 1993). Antigen-deficient cells which survive after treatment with a single IT were killed when that IT was combined with a second or third IT directed against a different antigen on the same cell.

IT cocktails consisting of ITs against CD25, CD30, and IRac (70kDa) on L540 Hodgkin's cells in any combination have demonstrated superior anti-tumor activity to single ITs, both in vitro and when used to treat solid human Hodgkin's tumors in nude mice (ENGERT et al. 1995). In SCID mice bearing disseminated Daudi lymphomas, an IT cocktail consisting of HD37 (anti-CD19)-dgA and RFB4 (anti-CD22)-dgA was shown to kill an equivalent of 5 logs of tumor cells, while HD37-dgRTA alone killed 2 logs and RFB4-dgRTA alone killed 4 logs (GHETIE et al. 1992). Studies in nude mice have reported superior effects of IT cocktails against non-T leukemia cells with ITs against CALLA (SN5-A) and a leukemia-associated surface glycoprotein (SN6-A) (HARA et al. 1988).

3 Clinical Trials with Ricin A-Chain Immunotoxins

3.1 Anti-CD5-Ricin A-Chain

Initial studies with RTA-based ITs in non-Hodgkin's lymphoma examined RTA conjugated to the Moab anti-CD5. This construct produced four partial responses in 14 patients with cutaneous T cell lymphoma (LeMaistre et al. 1991). The dominant toxicity was the occurrence of vascular leak syndrome (VLS) and reversible hepatic dysfunction. The latter was most likely due to the localization of the IT in the liver, since the RTA was fully glycosylated.

3.2 Anti-breast Cancer Immunotoxin 260F9-rRTA

When recombinant RTA was conjugated to the anti-breast carcinoma cell antibody 260F9 and used in patients with advanced breast cancer, VLS dominated the toxicity profile (Weiner et al. 1989). In addition, a neurologic syndrome consisting of sensorimotor neuropathy complicated the use of this agent. This unexpected side effect was ultimately linked to an unsuspected cross-reaction of the antibody with a determinant on either Schwann cells or myelin (Gould et al. 1989).

3.3 Anti-B Cell Immunotoxins RFB4-dgRTA and HD 37-dgRTA

The CD22 and CD19 determinants, expressed on adult B cell lymphomas, have been targeted in a series of clinical studies using dgRTA ITs. The Fab' fragment of the CD22-directed antibody RFB4 was linked to dgRTA and the resulting IT was studied in a regimen involving bolus doses administered every 48h for up to six doses. Partial remissions (PRs) of 1–4 months duration were noted in 38% of 15 patients, and VLS was the dominant reversible toxicity. Expressive aphasia and rhabdomyolysis were dose limiting toxicities. The $T_{1/2}$ of the IT was short, as can be expected for a relatively small molecule (Vitetta et al. 1991). A similarly designed phase-I trial using bolus administration of the RFB4-dgRTA in its IgG form gave five PRs and one complete remission (CR) lasting 30–78 days in 26 patients. VLS was the dose-limiting toxicity (Amlot et al. 1993). In addition, there was a trend toward decreased toxicity in patients with evidence of bulky disease including splenomegaly. The most prominent clinical trials in lymphoma patients are summarized in Table 3.

In an effort to reduce the incidence of VLS, a phase-I trial using a continuous infusion regimen was conducted (Sausville et al. 1995). In this trial, the IT was administered continuously over 192h (8 days). Despite this, there was essentially no difference in the maximal tolerated dose (MTD; 19mg/m^2 per 8 days) compared to the intermittent bolus dosing schedule. This study therefore concluded that there was no improvement in therapeutic index by administering the IT as a continuous infusion. The RFB4-dgRTA construct showed evidence of clinical activity, with four of 16 evaluable patients achieving PRs. The highest serum concentrations (> 1000ng/ml) on days 2 or 3 of the infusion were predictive of severe VLS. This observation was the first clear evidence of a relationship between the IT concentration in the blood and the occurrence of VLS. The $T_{1/2}$ of the IT was also variable, ranging as high as 23h in certain patients. Small numbers of circulating tumor cells, detectable in some cases only by flow cytometric analyses, correlated

Table 3. Clinical trials with ricin A-chain immunotoxins in lymphoma patients

Disease	Antigen	Toxin	Application	Toxicity	Immunogenicity	Response	Reference
B-NHL	CD22	Fab' RFB4-dgRTA	4 h infusion Day 1-3-5-7	VLS, myalgia, rhabdomyolysis	1/14 HAMA 4/14 HARA	5/14 PR	Vitetta et al. 1991
B-NHL	CD22	RFB4-SMPT-dgRTA	4 h infusion Day 1-3-5-7	VLS, myalgia, rhabdomyolysis	7/26 HAMA 8/26 HARA	1/26 CR; 5/26 PR	Amlot et al. 1993
B-NHL	CD22	RFB4-SMPT-dgRTA	Continuous infusion Day 1-8	VLS	5/15 HAMA 6/15 HARA	4/16 PR	Sausville et al. 1995
B-NHL	CD19	IgG-HD37-dgRTA	4 h infusion Day 1-3-5-7	VLS, aphasia, rhabdomyolysis, acrocyanosis	4/15 HAMA 5/15 HARA	1/23 CR; 1/23 PR	Stone et al. 1996
B-NHL	CD19	IgG-HD37-dgRTA	Continuous infusion Day 1-8	VLS, acrocyanosis	2/8 HAMA 2/8 HARA	1/9 PR	Stone et al. 1996
B-NHL	CD19	IgG-HD37- dgRTA	4 h infusion Day 1-3-5-7	VLS, myalgia, rhabdomyolysis	2/7 HAMA/HARA	1/8 PR	Conry et al. 1995
Hodgkin's lymphoma	CD25	IgG-RFT5- dgRTA	4 h infusion Day 1-3-5-7	VLS, fatigue, myalgia	6/15 HAMA 7/15 HARA	2/15 PR	Engert et al. 1997

NHL, non-Hodgkin's lymphoma; VLS, vascular leak syndrome; HAMA, human anti-mouse antibodies; HARA, human anti-ricin antibodies; CR, complete remission; PR, partial remission.

with decreased toxicity. These patients also tended to have increased volumes of distribution (Vd) of the IT with lower circulating IT levels achieved during the infusion. A notable trend using both the bolus and continuous infusion regimens was the likelihood of a better clinical response in patients with smaller tumor burdens ($< 100 cm^2$), reinforcing the potential value of this IT in patients with minimal disease.

A major problem in the use of anti-CD22-directed ITs is the variable expression of CD22 even on cells within the same tumor, and the fact that at best only 65%–70% of tumors are CD22+. In contrast, the CD19 determinant is more ubiquitously expressed on cells in adult lymphoid tumors. The anti-CD19-Moab HD37 was therefore used to construct HD37-dgRTA, and this agent was studied in regimens involving both intermittent bolus and continuous infusion. Although this IT was not as cytotoxic as RFB4-dgRTA, it was still highly potent. When given as an intermittent bolus infusion every 48 h for four doses, the MTD was $16 mg/m^2$ per 8 days. VLS again defined the MTD, and rhabdomyolysis was the dose-limiting toxicity, encountered at $24 mg/m^2$ per 8 days. Using the continuous-infusion regimen, the MTD again was $19.2 mg/m^2$ per 8 days, which is very comparable to the MTD using the bolus regimen. Of 32 evaluable patients from both bolus and continuous infusion regimens, there was one persisting CR (> 40 months) and two PRs (STONE et al. 1996). Of interest, when the dose of IT was administered in a regimen (four doses at 4h intervals) designed to produced sustained serum concentrations for 36h, there was apparent augmentation of toxicity, with an increased tendency for VLS and an MTD of only $8 mg/m^2$ (CONRY et al. 1995). Peak serum levels were highest in patients experiencing the greatest toxicity, as expected from prior experience with dgRTA ITs.

A novel, but infrequent, toxicity encountered with dgRTA ITs was reversible distal digital acrocyanosis, resembling a protracted vasoconstrictor phase of Raynaud's phenomenon. This could not be explained on the basis of circulating immune complexes or evidence of active inflammatory vasculitis and was observed in patients on both the continuous and the bolus infusion schedules (STONE et al. 1996).

Based on preclinical models in the SCID-Daudi system of disseminated lymphoma, a cocktail of ITs both in early stage and advanced diseases would be expected to augment the response compared to either of the ITs alone. Accordingly, a phase-I trial of a 1:1 mixture of the RFB4-dgRTA and HD37-dgRTA ITs (Combotox) is currently being completed. Initial results suggest that the MTD of Combotox in patients with low tumor burdens with no circulating tumor cells will be $10 mg/m^2$ per 8 days of total IT, with VLS defining the MTD; the MTD will be higher in patients with circulating tumor cells. This finding underscores a major difference for ITs as compared to more usual cancer chemotherapeutic agents; the MTD is a function of tumor burden and possibly site of disease. Of 19 evaluable patients thus far entered on the Combotox protocol, there has been one PR and four minor responses or stable disease. Combotox was well tolerated at $10 mg/m^2$. This regimen is now being considered in conjunction with chemotherapy in a minimal disease setting, in which Combotox is administered to patients after prior "debulking" with combination chemotherapy.

3.4 Anti-CD25-dgRTA

The anti-CD25 IT RFT5-dgRTA was used in a phase-I dose escalation trial in patients with refractory Hodgkin's lymphoma. The IT was constructed by linking the Moab RFT5 via SMPT to dg RTA (ENGERT et al. 1990a). All patients in this trial had advanced disease with massive tumor burdens and were heavily pretreated. The IT was administered i.v. over 4h on days 1, 3, 5, 7 for total doses of 5, 10, 15, or 20mg/m^2. Patients received one to four courses of treatment. The serum half life of the IT ranged from 4.0 to 10.5h. Side effects were related to VLS, i.e., decrease in serum albumin, edema, weight gain, hypotension, tachycardia, myalgia and weakness. At 15mg/m^2 one patient experienced a grade 3 myalgia. All three patients receiving the 20mg/m^2 dose showed NCI grade 3 toxicities (edema, nausea, dyspnea or tachycardia) and one patient had NCI grade 4 myalgia. Responses included two partial remissions (PR), one minor response (MR), three stable diseases (SD) and nine progressive diseases (PD). The maximal tolerated dose was 15mg/m^2 (ENGERT et al. 1997).

3.5 Vascular Leak Syndrome

Vascular leak syndrome refers to hypoalbuminemia and edema in patients without intrinsic cardiac, renal or hepatic disease. It has many etiologies including sepsis, high dose cytokine treatment and, in our experience, IT treatment. The common pathophysiologic mechanism appears to be alterations of endothelial cell permeability. A surprising outcome of initial clinical trials using both ricin-based and *Pseudomonas* exotoxin-based ITs is that both produced VLS as the dose-limiting toxicity. This syndrome had previously been identified as an adverse effect following interleukin (IL)-2 therapy (ROSENSTEIN et al. 1986) and, therefore, initial speculations centered on the elaboration of cytokines to explain VLS after exposure to RTA-ITs. Efforts to document increases in IL-1, IL-2, IL-6, as well as circulating cell adhesion molecules during IT-induced VLS have, however, failed (SAUSVILLE et al. 1995). Tumor necrosis factor (TNF) levels did, however, increase in patients with more severe VLS (BALUNA et al. 1996). Mild VLS may be manifested as decreased urinary sodium excretion and asymptomatic hypoalbuminemia (SAUSVILLE et al. 1995). In its most severe form, it can result in pulmonary edema with respiratory insufficiency and accumulation of massive pleural and pericardial effusions (VITETTA et al. 1991; AMLOT et al. 1993; SAUSVILLE et al. 1995; STONE et al. 1996; CONRY et al. 1995). The relationship between VLS and rhabdomyolysis to azotemia or reversible aphasia in the absence of underlying fixed brain lesions (also encountered at the highest dose levels of ricin-derived ITs) is unclear. Since the above side effects are never seen without concomitant VLS, they perhaps represent extreme manifestations of VLS in skeletal muscle and brain, respectively.

Recent evidence indicates that VLS is a nontargeted toxic effect of these toxins. RTA can directly damage vascular endothelial cells, which can then lead to an increase in surrogate assays for permeability in tissue culture (SOLER-RODRIGUEZ et al. 1993). The mechanism underlying this effect has recently been proposed to be due to the binding of RTA to fibronectin, thus preventing it from binding to its receptors on endothelial cells and causing cell damage. This has led to the suggestion that exogenously administered fibronectin may retard the occurrence of VLS (BALUNA et al. 1995). There is also a correlation between the peak serum concentration of IT achieved and the occurrence of VLS (SAUSVILLE et al. 1995), suggesting that prospective pharmacologic monitoring of serum levels of IT in conjunction with fibronectin levels may facilitate dose adjustments which will decrease the incidence or severity of VLS. Prophylactic steroids (SIEGALL et al. 1994) are also being evaluated in an effort to decrease the incidence of VLS but their efficacy has not been demonstrated in humans. An alternative mechanism for IT-mediated VLS in the case of *Pseudomonas*-derived toxins is the interaction of the targeting antibody with low-level expression of the targeting determinant on endothelial cells (KUAR et al. 1996). Irrespective of the mechanism of uptake, it is clear that adventitious exposure of endothelial cells to internalized ITs explains the occurrence of VLS.

3.6 Human Anti-immunotoxin Antibodies

The development of human anti-IT antibodies has been reported in most of the phase I/II trials thus far conducted. HAMAs (human anti-mouse antibody), HARAs (human anti-ricin antibody), or HACAs (anti-chimeric-antibody) can neutralize circulating ITs in the bloodstream of the patient resulting in a decreased half-life and in inefficient tumor cell killing. Higher titers of anti-IT antibodies can also cause allergic reactions. Attempts to reduce HAMA or HACA formation in humans including the coadministration of immunosuppressive agents have been unsuccessful so far. New drugs, including 15-deoxyspergualine (PAI et al. 1990), anti-RTA (BYERS et al. 1993), anti-CD4 (JIN et al. 1991) or CTLAIg (LINSLEY et al. 1992), are currently under investigation in clinical trials. Other promising approaches include the deletion of certain immunodominant epitopes on the toxin moiety and the use of humanized antibodies or mouse single chains lacking the Fc portion of the Moab. Antibodies consisting of human constant regions and murine variable or hypervariable regions have been generated using recombinant DNA technology (RIECHMANN et al. 1988). Totally "humanized" antibodies can be produced by targeted selection utilizing phage display (BARBAS et al. 1993).

4 Perspectives

4.1 New Immunotoxins

Over the past few years, new ITs generated by the chemical conjugation of RTA to different Moabs have been prepared and tested in vitro. The results have demonstrated that RTA-containing ITs directed against common B chronic lymphoblastic leukemia (CLL) antigen (FAGUET and AGEE 1993), B pre-lymphocytic leukemia (PLL), NHL (OKAZAKI et al. 1993), and human small-cell lung cancer (SCLC) (DERBYSHIRE et al. 1992,1996; DERBYSHIRE and WAWRZYNCZAK 1992) make effective ITs against their respective target cells. A construct containing RTA chemically linked to recombinant F(ab)2 anti-CD5 antibody was unexpectedly more active in vitro than its counterpart prepared with IgG (BETTER et al. 1993). An IT containing anti-CD25 antibody and dg RTA was used to eliminate activated CD25+ HIV-infected cells and to inhibit viral production (BELL et al. 1993). RTA has also been coupled to a bispecific antibody (anti-CD22/anti-CD3) and this IT was three- to 17-fold more cytotoxic to targeted CD22+ Daudi cells than its unconjugated counterpart in the presence of CD3+ effector lymphokine-activated killer T (LAK-T) cells (SHEN et al. 1994). In addition, ITs containing two as opposed to one RTA have been demonstrated to be more effective in vitro (GHETIE et al. 1995). A RTA-diphtheria toxin hybrid was more effective than conjugates prepared with either toxin alone (LI and RAMAKRISHNAN 1994).

4.2 Vascular Targeting

Although lymphomas have been successfully treated with ITs, epithelial (solid) tumors are less amenable to IT therapy (BYERS and BALDWIN 1988). This is because solid tumors are relatively large and poorly vascularized so that ITs do not penetrate the tumors very effectively (EPENETOS et al. 1986; SUNG et al. 1993). It has been proposed that an IT should be targeted to the dividing vascular endothelial cells (ECs) rather than the tumor cells themselves (DENEKAMP 1984). In this way, tumor cell heterogeneity will not be a problem, and one can kill the tumor by starving the cells of necessary nutrients and oxygen (DENEKAMP 1990). In addition, ECs are accessible, and, because they are normal cells, their antigens are unlikely to mutate. Furthermore, these ITs should be useful for treating a variety of tumors, because the destruction of a single blood vessel should result in the death of a large number of tumor cells.

One example of the potential efficacy of the vascular targeting approach was reported recently using a solid neuroblastoma model in mice. The tumor cells had been transfected with a mouse interferon (IFN)-γ gene resulting in a substantial up-regulation of class-II antigens on the blood vessels of the tumor. A single intravenous injection of an anti-class-II RTA IT into mice bearing large neuroblastoma tumors caused complete thrombosis of the tumor vasculature, wide-spread infarction, and dramatic tumor regression (BURROWS and THORPE 1993).

The future success of vascular targeting depends on defining unique antigens on dividing or activated but not resting ECs. Surface markers such as EN7/44, endoglin (CD105), endosialin, and E-9 Ag are possible candidates for vascular targeting.

4.3 Treatment of Minimal Residual Disease

Minimal residual disease (MRD) is defined as any tumor cell surviving intensive therapy (HAGENBEEK and MARTENS 1989). Clinical trials in lymphoma patients showed a strong correlation between MRD and poor outcome (GRIBBEN et al. 1991; SHARP et al. 1992; CAMPANA and PUI 1995). Since residual lymphoma cells are very likely to cause clinical relapses, the long-term goal for curing leukemias and lymphomas is the elimination of these cells. One prerequisite for the investigation into MRD was the development of new techniques such as fluorescent in situ hybridization with chromosome-specific probes (FISH) (CUNEO et al. 1992) or multicolor FACS analysis (CAMPANA et al. 1991) detecting occult tumor cells which cannot be monitored by standard histochemistry. Clonogenic assays are also well suited for detecting proliferating residual tumor cells in bone marrow and peripheral blood (SHARP et al. 1992). Finally, residual tumor cells can be investigated by polymerase chain reaction (PCR) with very high sensitivity (DREXLER et al. 1995).

MRD should be the ideal target for IT therapy since tumor burdens are small and cell clusters are well vascularized. However, to date, most clinical trials conducted with ITs have been performed in heavily pretreated patients with large tumor burdens. The best approach for using ITs in humans would be in an adjuvant setting together with or shortly after conventional treatment. A first, randomized, clinical phase-III trial (GROSSBARD et al. 1993) has been completed in patients with B cell NHL after high-dose chemotherapy and subsequent stem cell transplantation using a blocked ricin IT against CD19 (anti-B4-bR). Similar phase-II studies with a combination of HD37-dgRTA and RFB4-dgRTA will commence soon.

5 Summary

Since MRD is the major cause for relapses of malignant diseases, strategies utilizing ITs to target tumor cells surviving conventional treatment have attracted scientific and clinical interest. Many different ITs against various blood-borne as well as solid malignancies have demonstrated specific potent anti-tumor effects in vitro and in animal models. Some of these have already undergone clinical phase I/II-trials. The dose-limiting toxicities of RTA ITs include manifestation of VLS presenting as decreased urinary sodium excretion, hypoalbuminemia, fatigue, hypotonia, myalgia, pulmonary edema, or rhabdomyolysis. Problems encountered clinically include the development of HAMA, HARA, and HACA and the selection of antigen-deficient malignant clones. Most clinical trials performed with ITs so far were conducted in heavily pretreated patients presenting with high tumor burdens. Thus, the responses observed with ITs in these trials are very encouraging and warrant further exploration.

Acknowledgements. This work was supported in part by the Deutsche Forschungsgemeinschaft, Grant Di 184/9–7, TP9, the Deutsche Krebshilfe, Grant W125/94/En 2 and NIH Grant CA28149. We thank Ms. C. Self for secretarial assistance.

References

Amlot PL, Stone MJ, Cunningham D, Fay J, Newman J, Collins R, May R, McCarthy M, Richardson J, Ghetie V et al (1993) A Phase I study of an anti-CD22-deglycosylated ricin A-chain immunotoxin in the treatment of B-cell lymphomas resistant to conventional therapy. Blood 82:2624–2633

Baluna R, Getie V, Oppenhimer-Marks N, Vitetta ES (1995) The binding of ricin A-chain immunotoxin to fibronectin: possible implications for vascular leak syndrome in immunotoxin-treated patients. 4th international symposium on immunotoxins, p 144

Baluna R, Sausville EA, Stone MJ, Stetler-Stevenson MA, Uhr J, Vitetta ES (1996) Decreases in levels of serum fibronectin predict the severity of vascular leak syndrome in patients treated with ricin A-chain-containing immunotoxins. Clin Cancer Res 2:1705–1712

Barbas CF III, Amberg W, Simonesits A et al (1993) Selection of human anti-hapten antibodies from semisynthetic libraries. Gene 137:57–62

Bell KD, Ramilo O, Vitetta ES (1993) Combined use of an immunotoxin and cyclosporine to prevent both activated and quiescent peripheral blood T cells from producing type 1 human immunodeficiency virus. Proc Natl Acad Sci USA 90:1411–1415

Better M, Bernhard SL, Lei SP, Fishwild DM, Lane JA, Carroll SF, Horwitz AH (1993) Potent anti-cd5 ricin-A-chain immunoconjugates from bacterially produced fab' and f(ab')2. Proc Natl Acad Sci USA 90:457–461

Bjorn MJ, Ring D, Frankel A (1985) Evaluation of monoclonal antibodies for the development of breast cancer immunotoxins. Cancer Res 45:1214–1221

Blakey DC, Thorpe PE (1988) An overview of therapy with immunotoxins containing ricin or its A-chain. Antibody Immunoconj Radiopharm 1:1–16

Blakey DC, Watson GJ, Knowles PP, Thorpe PE (1987) Effect of chemical deglycosylation of ricin A-chain on the in vivo fate and cytotoxic activity of an immunotoxin composed of ricin A-chain and anti-Thy 1.1 antibody. Cancer Res 47:947–952

Blakey DC, Skilleter DN, Price RJ, Thorpe PE (1988) Uptake of native and deglycosylated ricin A-chain immunotoxins by mouse liver parenchymal and non-parenchymal cells in vitro and in vivo. Biochim Biophys Acta 968:172–178

Bourrie BJ, Casellas P, Blythman HE, Jansen FK (1986) Study of the plasma clearance of antibody–ricin-A-chain immunotoxins. Evidence for specific recognition sites on the A-chain that mediate rapid clearance of the immunotoxin. Eur J Biochem 155:1–10

Burrows FJ, Thorpe PE (1993) Eradication of large solid tumors in mice with an immunotoxin directed against tumor vasculature. Proc Natl Acad Sci USA 90:8996–9000

Byers VS, Baldwin RW (1988) Therapeutic strategies with monoclonal antibodies and immunoconjugates. Immunology 65:329–335

Byers VS, Pimm MV, Pawluczyk I, Lee HM, Scannon PJ, Baldwin RW (1987) Biodistribution of ricin toxin A-chain monoclonal antibody 79IT/36 immunotoxins and the influence of heptic blocking agents. Cancer Res 47:5277–5283

Byers VS, Austin EB, Clegg JA et al (1993) Suppression of antibody responses to ricin A chain (RTA) by monoclonal anti-RTA antibodies. J Clin Immunol 13:406–412

Campana D, Pui CH (1995) Detection of minimal residual disease in acute leukemia: methodologic advances and clinical significance. Blood 85:1416–1434

Campana D, Coustan-Smith E, Behm FG (1991) The definition of remission in acute leukemia with immunologic methods. Bone Marrow Transplant 8:429–437

Casellas P, Jansen FK (1988) Immunotoxin enhancers. In: Frankel AE (ed) Immunotoxins. Kluwer Academic, Norwell, pp 351–371

Casellas P, Bourrie BJP, Gros P, Jansen F (1984) Kinetics of cytotoxicity induced by immunotoxins. Enhancement by lysosomotropic amines and carboxylic ionophores. J Biol Chem 259:9359–9364

Conry RM, Khazaeli MB, Saleh MN, Ghetie V, Vitetta ES, Liu TP, Lobuglio AF (1995) Phase I trial of an anti-CD19 deglycosylated ricin A-chain immunotoxin in non-Hodgkin's lymphoma: effect of an intensive schedule of administration. J Immunother 18(4):231–241

Cumber AJ, Forrester JA, Foxwell BM, Ross WC, Thorpe PE (1985) Preparation of antibody-toxin conjugates. Methods Enzymol 112:207–225

Cuneo A, Wlodarska I, Sayed AM, Piva N, Carli MG, Fagioli F, Tallarico A, Pazzi I, Ferrari L, Cassiman J et al. (1992) Non-radioactive in situ hybridization for the detection and monitoring of trisomy 12 in B-cell chronic lymphocytic leukaemia. Br J Haematol 81:192–196

Denekamp J (1984) Vasculature as a target for tumor therapy. Prog Appl Microcirc 4:28–38

Denekamp J (1990) Vascular attack as a therapeutic strategy for cancer. Cancer Metastasis Rev 9:267–282

Derbyshire EJ, Wawrzynczak EJ (1992) An antimucin immunotoxin bre-3-ricin A-chain is potently and selectively toxic to human small-cell lung cancer. Int J Cancer 52:624–630

Derbyshire EJ, Stahel RA, Wawrzynczak EJ (1992) Cytotoxic properties of a ricin A-chain immunotoxin recognizing the cluster-5 A antigen associated with human small-cell lung cancer. Cancer Immunol Immunother 35:417–420

Derbyshire EJ, Henry RV, Stahel RA, Wawrzynczak EJ (1996) Potent cytotoxic action of the immunotoxin SWA11-ricin A-chain against human small lung cancer cell lines. Br J Cancer 66:444–451

Drexler HG, Borkhardt A, Janssen JW (1995) Detection of chromosomal translocations in leukemia-lymphoma cells by polymerase chain reaction. Leuk Lymphoma 19:359–380

Engert A, Burrows F, Jung W, Tazzari PL, Stein H, Pfreundschuh M, Diehl V, Thorpe P (1990a) Evaluation of ricin A-chain-containing immunotoxins directed against the CD30 antigen as potential reagents for the treatment of Hodgkin's disease. Cancer Res 50:84–88

Engert A, Martin G, Pfreundschuh M, Amlot P, Hsu SM, Diehl V, Thorpe P (1990b) Anti-tumor effects of ricin A-chain immunotoxins from intact antibodies and Fab' fragments on solid human Hodgkin's disease tumors in mice. Cancer Res 50:2929–2935

Engert A, Gottstein C, Bohlen H, Winkler U, Schön G, Manske O, Schnell R, Diehl V, Thorpe P (1995) Cocktails composed of ricin A-chain immunotoxins against different antigens on Hodgkin and Sternberg-Reed (H-RS) cells have superior anti-tumor effects against H-RS cells in vitro and solid Hodgkin's tumors in mice. Int J Cancer 63:304–309

Engert A, Diehl V, Schnell R, Radszuhn A, Hatwig M, Drillich S, Schön G, Bohlen H, Tesch H, Hansmann M, Barth S, Schindler J, Ghetie V, Uhr J, Vitetta E (1997) A Phase-I study of an anti-CD25 ricin A-chain immunotoxin (RFT5-SMPT-dgA) in patients with refractory Hodgkin's lymphoma. Blood 1: 403–410

Epenetos AA, Snok D, Durbin H, Johnson PM, Taylor-Papadimitriou J (1986) Limitations of radiolabeled monoclonal antibodies for localization of human neoplasms. Cancer Res 46:3183–3191

Faguet GB, Agee JF (1993) Four ricin chain a-based immunotoxins directed against the common chronic lymphocytic leukemia antigen – invitro characterization. Blood 82:536–543

Frankel AE, Ring DB, Tringale F, Hsieh-Ma ST (1985) Tissue distribution of breast cancer-associated antigens defined by monoclonal antibodies. J Biol Resp Modif 4:273–286

Fulton RJ, Blakey DC, Knowles PP, Uhr JW, Thorpe PE, Vitetta ES (1986) Production of ricin A1, A2, and B chains and characterization of their toxicity. J Biol Chem 261:5314–5319

Fulton RJ, Tucker TF, Vitetta ES, Uhr JW (1988a) Pharmacokinetics of tumor-reactive immunotoxins in tumor-bearing mice: effect of antibody valency and deglycosylation of the ricin A-chain on clearance and tumor localization. Cancer Res 48:2618–2625

Fulton RJ, Uhr JW, Vitetta ES (1988b) In vivo therapy of the BCL1 tumor: effect of immunotoxin valency and deglycosylation of the ricin A-chain. Cancer Res 48:2626–2631

Ghetie M, May RD, Till M, Uhr JW, Ghetie V, Knowles PP, Relf M, Brown A, Wallace PM, Janossy G et al (1988) Evaluation of ricin A-chain-containing immunotoxins directed against CD19 and CD22 antigens on normal and malignant human B-cells as potential reagents for in vivo therapy. Cancer Res 48:2610–2617

Ghetie M, Tucker K, Richardson J, Uhr JW, Vitetta ES (1992) The anti-tumor activity of an anti-CD22 immunotoxin in SCID mice with disseminated Daudi lymphoma is enhanced by either an anti-CD19 antibody or an anti-CD19 immunotoxin. Blood 80:2315–2320

Ghetie M-A, Tucker K, Richardson J, Uhr JW, Vitetta ES (1994) Eradication of minimal disease in severe combined immunodeficient mice with disseminated Daudi lymphoma using chemotherapy and an immunotoxin cocktail. Blood 84:702–707

Ghetie V, Engert A, Schnell R, Vitetta ES (1995) The in vivo anti-tumor activity of immunotoxins containing two versus one deglycosylated ricin A chains. Cancer Lett 98:97–101

Ghetie MA, Podar EM, Gordon BE, Pantazis P, Uhr JW, Vitetta ES (1996) Combination immunotoxin treatment and chemotherapy in SCID mice with advanced, disseminated Daudi lymphoma. Int J Cancer 68:93–96

Gould BJ, Borowitz MJ, Groves ES, Carter PW, Anthony D, Weiner LM, Frankel AE (1989) Phase I study of an anti-breast cancer immunotoxin by continuous infusion: report of a targeted toxic effect not predicted by animal studies. J Natl Cancer Inst 81:775–781

Gros O, Gros P, Jansen FK, Vidal H (1985) Biochemical aspects of immunotoxin preparation. J Immunol Methods 81:283–297

Grossbard ML, Gribben JG, Freedman AS et al (1993) Adjuvant immunotoxin therapy with anti-B4-blocked ricin after autologous bone marrow transplantation for patients with B-cell non-Hodgkin's lymphoma. Blood 81:2263–2271

Gribben JG, Freedman AS, Woo SD et al (1991) All advanced stage non-Hodgkin's lymphomas with a polymerase chain reaction amplifiable breakpoint of bcl-2 have residual cells containing the bcl-2 rearrangement at evaluation and after treatment. Blood 78:3275–3280

Hagenbeek A, Martens ACM (1989) Cryopreservation of autologous marrow grafts in acute leukemia: survival of in vivo clonogenic leukemic cells and normal hematopoietic stem cells. Leuk 3:535–537

Hara H, Luo Y, Haruta Y, Seon BK (1988) Efficient transplantation of human non-T-leukemia cells into nude mice and induction of complete regression of the transplanted distinct tumors by ricin A-chain conjugates of monoclonal antibodies SN5 and SN6. Cancer Res 48:4673–4680

Jansen B, Vallera DA, Jaszcz WB, Nguyen D, Kersey JH (1992) Successful treatment of human acute T-cell leukemia in SCID mice using the anti-CD7-deglycosylated ricin A-chain immunotoxin DA7. Cancer Res 52:1314–1321

Jansen FK, Blythman HE, Carriere D, Casellas P, Diaz J, Gros P, Hennequin JR, Paolucci F, Pau B, Poncelet P et al (1980) High specific cytotoxicity of antibody-toxin hybrid molecules (immunotoxins) for target cells. Immunol Lett 2:97–102

Jansen FK, Blythman HE, Carriere D, Casellas P, Gros O, Gros P, Laurent JC, Paolucci F, Pau B, Poncelet P et al (1982) Immunotoxins: hybrid molecules combining high specificity and potent cytotoxicity. Immunol Rev 62:185–216

Jin FS, Youle RJ, Johnson VG et al (1991) Suppression of the immune response to immunotoxins with anti-CD4 monoclonal antibodies. J Immunol 146:1806–1811

Katre NV (1993) The conjugation of proteins with polyethylene glycol and other polymers. Adv Drug Delivery Rev 10:91–114

Kimura Y, Hase S, Kobayashi Y, Kyogoku Y, Ikenaka T, Funatsu G (1988) Structures of sugar chains of ricin D. J Biochem (Tokyo) 103:944–949

Kitamura K, Takahashi T, Yamaguchi T, Noguchi A, Takashina K, Tsurumi H, Inagake M, Toyokuni T, Hakomori S (1991) Chemical engineering of the monoclonal antibody A7 by polyethylene glycol for targeting cancer chemotherapy. Cancer Res 51:4310–4315

Kitamura K, Takahashi T, Takashina K, Yamaguchi T, Noguchi A, Tsurumi H, Tojokuni T, Hakomori S (1996) Polyethylene glycol modification of the monoclonal antibody A7 enhances its tumor localization. Biochem Biophys Res Commun 171:1387–1394

Knowles PP, Thorpe PE (1987) Purification of immunotoxins containing ricin A-chain and abrin A-chain using Blue Sepharose CL-6B. Anal Biochem 160:440–443

Kuar G, Pai LM, Pastan I (1996) Immunotoxins targeting Le4 damage human endothelial cells in an antibody specific mode: reliance to vascular leak syndrome. 4th international symposium on immunotoxins, p 115

Laman JD, Claassen E, Noelle RJ (1996) Functions of CD40 and its ligand, gp39 (CH40L). Crit Rev Immunol 16:59–108

Lamb FI, Roberts LM, Lord JM (1985) Nucleotide sequence of cloned cDNA coding for preproricin. Eur J Biochem 148:265–270

LeMaistre CF, Rosen S, Frankel A, Kornfeld S, Saria E, Meneghetti C, Drajesk J, Fishwild D, Scannon P, Byers V (1991) Phase I trial of H65-RTA immunoconjugate in patients with cutaneous T-cell lymphoma. Blood 78:1173–1182

Lenschow DJ, Walunas TL, Bluestone JA (1996) CD28/B7 system of T cell costimulation. Annu Rev Immunol 14:233–258

Li BY, Ramakrishnan S (1994) Recombinant hybrid toxin with dual enzymatic activities. Potential use in preparing highly effective immunotoxins. J Biol Chem 269(4):2652–2658

Linsley PS, Wallace PM, Johnson J et al (1992) Immunosuppression in vivo by a soluble form of the CTLA-4 T cell activation molecule. Science 257:792–795
Masuho Y, Kishida K, Saito M, Umeto N, Hara T (1982) Importance of the antigen-binding valency and the nature of cross-linking bond in ricin A-chain conjugates with antibody. J Biochem 91:1583–1591
May RD, Finkelman F, Uhr JW, Vitetta ES (1990) Evaluation of ricin A-chain-containing immunotoxins directed against different epitopes on the deltA-chain of sIgD on murine B cells. J Immunol 144:3637–3642
McIntosh DP, Edwards DC, Cumber AJ, Parnell GD, Dean CJ, Ross WC, Forrester JA (1983) Ricin B chain converts a non-cytotoxic antibody-ricin A-chain conjugate into a potent and specific cytotoxic agent. FEBS Lett 164:17–20
O'Hare M, Roberts LM, Thorpe PE, Watson GJ, Prior B, Lord JM (1987) Expression of ricin A-chain in *Escherichia coli*. FEBS Lett 216:73–78
O'Hare M, Brown AN, Hussain K, Gebhardt A, Watson G, Roberts LM, Vitetta ES, Thorpe PE, Lord JM (1990) Cytotoxicity of a recombinant ricin-A-chain fusion protein containing a proteolytical cleavable spacer sequence. FEBS Lett 273:200–204
Okazaki M, Luo Y, Han T, Yoshida M, Seon BK (1993) Three new monoclonal antibodies that define a unique antigen associated with prolymphocytic leukemia/non-Hodgkin's lymphoma and are effectively internalized after binding to the cell surface antigen. Blood 81:84–94
Pai LH, FitzGerald DJ, Tepper M et al (1990) Inhibition of antibody response to Pseudomonas exotoxin and an immunotoxin containing Pseudomonas exotoxin by 15-deoxyspergulin in mice. Cancer Res 50:7750–7753
Pantel K, Schlimok G, Braun S, Kutter D, Lindemann F, Schaller G, Funke I, Izbicki JR, Riethmüller G (1993) Differential expression of proliferation-associated molecules in individual micrometastatic carcinoma cells. J Natl Cancer Inst 85:1419–1424
Parham P (1983) On the fragmentation of monoclonal IgG1, IgG2a and IgG2b from BALB/c mice. J Immunol 131:2895–2902
Press OW, Vitetta ES, Farr AG, Hansen JA, Martin PJ (1986) Evaluation of ricin A-chain immunotoxins directed against human T cells. Cell Immunol 102:10–20
Press OW, Martin P, Thorpe PE, Vitetta ES (1988) Ricin A-chain containing immunotoxins directed against different epitopes on the CD2 molecule differ in their ability to kill normal and malignant T cells. J Immunol 141:4410–4417
Ramakrishnan S, Houston LL (1984a) Comparison of the selective cytotoxic effects of immunotoxins containing ricin A-chain or pokeweed antiviral protein and anti-Thy 1.1 monoclonal antibodies. Cancer Res 44:201–208
Ramakrishnan S, Houston LL (1984b) Inhibition of human acute lymphoblastic leukemia cells by immunotoxins: potentiation by chloroquine. Science 223:58–61
Ramakrishnan S, Bjorn MJ, Houston LL (1989) Recombinant ricin A-chain conjugated to monoclonal antibodies: improved tumor cell inhibition in the presence of lysosomotropic compounds. Cancer Res 49:613–617
Raso V (1988) Growth factors and other ligands. In: Frankel AE (ed) Immunotoxins. Kluwer Academic, Norwell, pp 297–323
Raso V, Griffin T (1980) Specific cytotoxicity of a human immunoglobulin directed Fab'-ricin A conjugate. J Immunol 125:2610–2616
Raso V, Lawrence J (1984) Carboxylic ionophores enhance the cytotoxic potency of ligand- and antibody-delivered ricin A-chain. J Exp Med 160:1234–1240
Riechmann L, Clark M, Waldmann H et al (1988) Reshaping human antibodies for therapy. Nature 332:323–327
Rosenstein M, Ettinghausen SE, Rosenberg SA (1986) Extravasation of vascular fluid mediated by the systemic administration of recombinant interleukin-2. J Immunol 137:1735–1742
Sausville EA, Headlee D, Stetler-Stevenson M, Jaffe ES, Solomon D, Figg WD, Herdt J, Kopp WC, Rager H, Steinberg SM et al (1995) Continuous infusion of the anti-CD22 immunotoxin, IgG-RFB4-SMPT-dgA in patients with B cell lymphoma: a phase I study. Blood 85:3457–3465
Sharp JG, Joshi SS, Armitage JO et al (1992) Significance of detection of occult non-Hodgkin's lymphoma in histologically uninvolved bone marrow by a culture technique. Blood 79:1074–1080
Shen G, Li J, Vitetta ES (1994) Bispecific anti-CD22/anti-CD3-ricin A-chain immunotoxin is cytotoxic to Daudi lymphoma cells but not T cells in vitro and shows both A-chain-mediated and LAK-T mediated killing. J Immunol 152:2368–2376

Shen G, Li J, Ghetie M, Ghetie V, May RD, Till M, Brown AN, Relf M, Knowles P, Uhr JW et al (1988) Evaluation of four CD22 antibodies as ricin A-chain-containing immunotoxins for the in vivo therapy of human B-cell leukemias and lymphomas. Int J Cancer 42:792–797

Siegall CB, Liggitt D, Chace D, Tepper MA, Fell HP (1994) Prevention of immunotoxin-mediated vascular leak syndrome in rats with retention of anti-tumor activity. Proc Natl Acad Sci USA 91(20):9514–9518

Siegall CB, Haggerty HG, Warner GL, Chace D, Mixan B, Linsley PS and Davidson T (1997) Prevention of immunotoxin-induced immunogenicity by coadministration with CTL41g enhances antitumor efficacy. J Immunol 159:5168–5173

Skilleter DN, Paine AJ, Stirpe F (1981) A comparison of the accumulation of ricin by hepatic parenchymal and non-parenchymal cells and its inhibition of protein synthesis. Biochim Biophys Acta 677:495–500

Smyth MJ, Pietersz GA, McKenzie IF (1987) Use of vasoactive agents to increase tumor perfusion and the anti-tumor efficacy of drug-monoclonal antibody conjugates. J Natl Cancer Inst 79:1367–1373

Soler-Rodriguez AM, Ghetie MA, Oppenheimer-Marks N, Uhr JW, Vitetta ES (1993) Ricin A-chain and ricin A-chain immunotoxins rapidly damage human endothelial cells: Implications for vascular leak syndrome. Exp Cell Res 206:227–239

Spooner RA, Allen DJ, Epenetos AA, Lord JM (1994) Expression of immunoglobulin heavy chain ricin A-chain fusions in mamalian cells. Mol Immunol 31:117–125

Stanworth DR, Turner MW (1978) Immunochemical analysis of immunoglobulins and their sub-units. In: Weir DM (ed) Handbook of experimental immunology. Blackwell Scientific, Oxford, pp 1–102

Stone MJ, Sausville EA, Fay JW, Headlee D, Collins RH, Figg WD, Stetler-Stevenson M, Jain V, Jaffe ES, Solomon D et al (1996) A phase I study of bolus versus continuous infusion of the anti-CD19 immunotoxin, IgG-HD-37-dgRTA, in patients with B-cell lymphoma. Blood 88(4):1188–1197

Sung C, Dedrick RL, Hall WA, Johnson PA, Youle RJ (1993) The spatial distribution of immunotoxins in solid tumors -assessment by quantitative autoradiography. Cancer Res 53:2092–2099

Svasti J, Milstein C (1972) The disulphide bridges of a mouse immunoglobulin G1 protein. Biochem J 126:837–850

Thorpe PE, Brown AN, Bremner JA Jr, Foxwell BM, Stirpe F (1985a) An immunotoxin composed of monoclonal anti-Thy 1.1 antibody and a ribosome-inactivating protein from Saponaria officinalis: potent anti-tumor effects in vitro and in vivo. J Natl Cancer Inst 75:151–159

Thorpe PE, Detre SI, Foxwell BMJ, Brown ANF, Skilleter DN, Wilson G, Forrester JA, Stirpe F (1985b) Modification of the carbohydrate in ricin with metaperiodate-cyanoborohydride mixtures. Effects on toxicity and in vivo distribution. Eur J Biochem 147:197–206

Thorpe PE, Blakey DC, Brown AN, Knowles PP, Knyba RE, Wallace PM, Watson GJ, Wawrzynczak EJ (1987a) Comparison of two anti-Thy 1.1-abrin A-chain immunotoxins prepared with different crosslinking agents: anti-tumor effects, in vivo fate, and tumor cell mutants. J Natl Cancer Inst 79:1101–1112

Thorpe PE, Wallace PM, Knowles PP, Relf MG, Brown ANF, Watson GJ, Knyba RE, Wawrzynczak EJ, Blakey DC (1987b) New coupling agents for the synthesis of immunotoxins containing a hindered disulfide bond with improved stability in vivo. Cancer Res 47:5924–5931

Thorpe PE, Wallace PM, Knowles PP, Relf MG, Brown ANF, Watson GJ, Blakey DC, Newell DR (1988) Improved anti-tumor effects of immunotoxins prepared with deglycosylated ricin A-chain and hindered disulfide linkages. Cancer Res 48:6396–6403

Till M, May RD, Uhr JW, Thorpe PE, Vitetta ES (1988) An assay that predicts the ability of monoclonal antibodies to form potent ricin A-chain-containing immunotoxins. Cancer Res 48:1119–1123

Vitetta ES, Cushley W, Uhr JW (1983) Synergy of ricin A-chain-containing immunotoxins and ricin B chain-containing immunotoxins in in vitro killing of neoplastic human B cells. Proc Natl Acad Sci USA 80:6332–6335

Vitetta ES, Fulton RJ, Uhr JW (1984) Cytotoxicity of a cell-reactive immunotoxin containing ricin A-chain is potentiated by an anti-immunotoxin containing ricin B chain. J Exp Med 160:341–346

Vitetta ES, Fulton RJ, May RD, Till M, Uhr JW (1987) Redesigning nature's poisons to create anti-tumor reagents. Science 238:1098–1104

Vitetta ES, Stone M, Amlot P, Fay J, May R, Till M, Newman J, Clark P, Collins R, Cunningham D et al (1991) A phase I immunotoxin trial in patients with B cell lymphoma. Cancer Res 51:4052–4058

Wawrzynczak EJ, Thorpe PE (1987) Methods for preparing immunotoxins: effects of the linkage on activity and stability. In: Vogel CW (ed) Immunoconjugates: antibody conjugates in radioimaging and therapy of cancer. Oxford University Press, New York, pp 28–55

Weiner LM, O'Dwyer J, Kitson J, Comis RL, Frankel AE, Bauer RJ, Konrad MS, Groves ES (1989) Phase I evaluation of an anti-breast carcinoma monoclonal antibody 260F9-recombinant ricin A-chain immunoconjugate. Cancer Res 49:4062–4067

Winkler U, Gottstein C, Schön G, Kapp U, Wolf J, Hansmann M-L, Bohlen H, Thorpe P, Diehl V, Engert A (1994) Successful treatment of disseminated human Hodgkin's disease in SCID mice with deglycosylated ricin A-chain immunotoxins. Blood 83:466–475

Youle RJ, Neville DM Jr (1982) Kinetics of protein synthesis inactivation by ricin-anti-Thy 1.1 monoclonal antibody hybrids. Role of the ricin-B subunit demonstrated by reconstitution. J Biol Chem 257:1598–1601

Clinical Trials with Blocked Ricin Immunotoxins

J.E. O'TOOLE[1], D. ESSELTINE[2], T.J. LYNCH[1], J.M. LAMBERT[2], and M.L. GROSSBARD[1]

1	Introduction	35
2	Ricin-Based Immunotoxins	36
3	Model Immunotoxins	38
4	Blocked Ricin Therapy of Hematologic Malignancies	38
4.1	Anti-B4-bR	41
4.1.1	Non-Hodgkin's Lymphoma	41
4.1.2	Chronic Lymphocytic Leukemia and Acute Lymphoblastic Leukemia	46
4.1.3	Multiple Myeloma	47
4.2	Anti-My9-bR	48
4.3	Anti-CD6-bR	50
5	Blocked Ricin Immunotoxin Therapy of Solid Tumors: N901-bR	50
6	Conclusions	53
References		54

1 Introduction

The use of combination chemotherapy and the introduction of new cytotoxic agents has resulted in therapeutic advances for patients with cancer. Unfortunately, even with the development of innovative multi-drug treatment regimens and the increasing availability of both autologous bone marrow transplantation (ABMT) and peripheral blood stem cell transplantation (PBSCT), the clinician lacks the necessary tools to successfully combat the progression of malignancy in the majority of patients. Furthermore, substantial morbidity and potential mortality is associated with the use of these aggressive treatment programs. New anti-tumor agents ideally should circumvent the two major limitations of current therapy: devastating nonspecific side effects and tumor cell resistance.

Immunotoxins (ITs) provide a theoretical solution to the aforementioned obstacles (VITETTA et al. 1987; GROSSBARD and NADLER 1992). By targeting specific

[1] Hematology-Oncology Unit, Massachusetts General Hospital, Cox 228, Boston, MA 02114, USA
[2] ImmunoGen, Inc., Cambridge, MA 02139, USA

antigens which reside on tumor cells alone (or tumor cells and an expendable population of normal cells), monoclonal antibodies (MoAbs) may deliver their toxic cargo to limited tissues, thereby avoiding systemic nonspecific toxicity. In addition, the cytotoxic mechanisms of most toxins conjugated to antibodies are decidedly different from those of conventional chemotherapeutic agents. Thus, conventional mechanisms of resistance may be bypassed.

Several protein toxins have been used in the IT therapy of cancer. These toxins are derived from both bacteria (diphtheria toxin, *Pseudomonas* exotoxin A) and plants (ricin, saporin, pokeweed anti-viral protein) and exert their cytotoxic effects by inhibiting protein synthesis. Molecular and biochemical manipulation of these toxins permits their conjugation to the MoAb of choice to target different malignancies while restricting their nonspecific toxicity.

One such modified toxin, blocked ricin (bR), has been conjugated to several MoAbs and studied already as a therapeutic agent in the treatment of non-Hodgkin's lymphoma (NHL), chronic lymphocytic leukemia (CLL), multiple myeloma (MM), acute lymphoblastic leukemia (ALL), acute myelogenous leukemia (AML), cutaneous T cell lymphoma (CTCL) and small cell lung cancer (SCLC). Phase I and II clinical trials have defined the maximum tolerated doses and dose-limiting toxicities of these agents. These bR-ITs have been administered, in most instances, with tolerable, reversible toxicities and have demonstrated biological activity in vivo. This chapter will describe the development and clinical use of four bR-ITs for the treatment of malignant disease.

2 Ricin-Based Immunotoxins

Blocked ricin ITs are composed of a MoAb and a modified ricin toxin which are chemically linked so that the active portion of the toxin will be liberated within the malignant cell but will not circulate free in the blood. Ricin, a heterodimeric protein derived from castor beans (*Ricinus communis*), consists of an A-chain and a B-chain (ENDO et al. 1987). When delivered at nanomolar or lower concentrations, ricin can kill more than 5 logs of both malignant and normal cells. Phase I clinical studies with native ricin suggested a maximum tolerated dose (MTD) of $23\mu g/m^2$, but the agent was not further developed for clinical use because of the absence of a therapeutic window due to high toxicity toward normal tissues (FODSTAD et al. 1984). If ricin were administered in its native state, this profound cytotoxicity would prove lethal to humans. The actual toxic moiety of ricin is the A-chain, which possesses N-glycosidase activity that inactivates the 60S ribosomal subunit. The enzymatic A-chain hydrolyzes an adenine-ribose linkage within the 23S rRNA, thereby halting protein synthesis (ENDO et al. 1987). The B-chain both binds nonspecifically to galactose residues present on the surface of all eukaryotic cells and facilitates translocation of the A-chain across the vesicular membrane into the cytosol after endocytosis of the entire protein. Linking ricin directly to a MoAb directed against a tumor-specific antigen will direct the toxin to tumor cells, but cannot avert nonspecific toxicity caused by binding of the B-chain.

A number of solutions have been proposed to alleviate the problems associated with nonspecific binding of the IT. One approach has been to isolate the ricin A-chain either by physical dissociation from the B-chain or by generation of a recombinant ricin molecule. Conjugation of ricin A-chain alone to a MoAb will eliminate the nonspecific binding capability of the conjugate. For example, VITETTA et al. (1991). have developed a conjugate between the RFB4 murine MoAb, which recognizes the CD22 antigen present on B cells, and deglycosylated ricin A-chain. By deglycosylating the A-chain through removal of mannose and fucose residues, nonspecific hepatic uptake of the IT can be minimized (BLAKEY et al. 1987). This IT has been administered to patients with B cell NHL with dose-limiting toxicities including pulmonary edema, expressive aphasia, and rhabdomyolysis. Notably, biological activity was observed in the form of five partial responses. Similarly, a conjugate has been developed between the H65 MoAb which targets the CD5 antigen and ricin A-chain (LeMAISTRE et al. 1991). This IT was used to treat patients with cutaneous T cell NHL, and partial responses again were seen. Side effects included edema, chills, fever, hypoalbuminemia, fatigue and myalgias. Despite the somewhat encouraging results of these studies, the obvious limitation with using isolated ricin A-chain toxins is that the translocation function of the B-chain is forfeited. Hence, the use of isolated ricin A-chain for developing ITs restricts the selection of MoAbs to those which have a capacity for internalization.

In an attempt to preserve the transport function of the B-chain, but to subvert its nonspecific binding capability, an altered ricin molecule has been synthesized in which the B-chain is covalently modified at the galactose-binding sites (LAMBERT et al. 1991a). The B-chain possesses two major binding sites for galactose although there is some evidence for at least one other, weaker, sugar-binding site (GOLDMACHER et al. 1992). Simple sugars bind with less affinity to the major binding sites on the B-chain than do more complex oligosaccharides. Therefore, modified glycopeptides containing N-linked oligosaccharides derived from fetuin have been constructed with terminal galactose residues available for binding and a reactive diclorotriazine moiety available for cross-linking to a protein. These affinity ligands adhere to the galactose binding sites and then become covalently attached to the B-chain, thus minimizing the galactose binding capability of ricin (LAMBERT et al. 1991b). This "blocked ricin" retains the translocation ability of the toxin. In vitro cytotoxicity studies of blocked ricin against Namalwa cells (a human B cell NHL cell line) demonstrate a 1000-fold reduction in the IC_{37} of blocked ricin vs native ricin. However, when a conjugate is made between blocked ricin and an anti-B cell MoAb, the full cytotoxic potential of native ricin against the targeted cell line is restored.

Future advances in the development of modified toxins are on the horizon. For example, it may be possible to produce a recombinant version of the ricin protein in which the galactose-binding regions of the ricin B-chain have been deleted while translocation capacity has been preserved. Such molecular manipulations offer the possibility of even greater reductions in nonspecific cytotoxicity.

3 Model Immunotoxins

Immunotoxins must meet certain criteria to be useful for clinical application (GROSSBARD and NADLER 1992). Among these are high specificity for the targeted antigen, high selectivity for the targeted population of cells, and demonstrated cytotoxic efficiency. The first and, in part, the second factors are mediated by the choice of MoAb and its target antigen. Rational antigens for IT targeting should: (1) be expressed on the clonogenic tumor cell; (2) be present at an adequate density on tumor cells to bind sufficient IT; (3) be absent from normal tissues or, in the case of hematological malignancies, be absent from hematopoietic stem cells; (4) not be shed into the circulation where the antigen can bind to IT and lead to its rapid clearance.

Tissue selectivity and potent cytotoxicity also are dependent on the choice of toxin. Blocked ricin does not demonstrate significant nonspecific binding to cells in vitro. In addition, when blocked ricin is conjugated to an antibody, sufficiently potent cytotoxicity is produced that the resultant IT can achieve a 3 log greater cell kill than conventional chemotherapy agents administered at tolerable doses. Blocked ricin has been conjugated to four different MoAbs for the treatment of cancer. The remainder of this chapter will discuss the clinical applications of these ITs for patients with neoplastic disease. We will attempt to provide some perspective on the tumors that have been treated to emphasize the dire need that exists to develop new therapeutic agents.

4 Blocked Ricin Immunotoxin Therapy of Hematologic Malignancies

Distinct advantages have been recognized in the application of IT therapy for the treatment of hematologic malignancy, in contrast to the treatment of solid tumors (GROSSBARD et al. 1992a). In the treatment of leukemia, lymphoma, and myeloma, lineage-specific antigens exist which can serve as appropriate targets for the IT. Moreover, tumor cells in these patients are relatively accessible to IT binding, although bulky fibrotic tumor masses seen in patients with NHL can limit IT diffusion and an abundance of circulating tumor cells can contribute to rapid IT clearance from serum. Because some of these malignancies are B cell in origin, the IT potentially may exert cytotoxicity towards normal B cells which may limit the development of human anti-mouse antibody (HAMA) and human anti-ricin antibody (HARA).

Clinical trials using three blocked ricin ITs (anti-B4-bR, anti-My9-bR, anti-CD6-bR) have been conducted in patients with NHL, CLL, MM, ALL, AML, and CTCL (Table 1). The majority of these studies were phase I clinical investigations designed to determine the maximum tolerated dose of IT and the toxicities of IT

Table 1. Clinical trials with blocked ricin immunotoxins

Immunotoxin	Disease	Phase	Patients (n)	MTD (total dose)	DLT (NCI CTC grade)	HAMA/HARA	Response
Anti-B4-bR	B-NHL, CLL, ALL	I	25	250μg/kg	Transaminase elevations (III)	9/25 HAMA 9/25 HARA	1 CR, 2 PR, 8 transient responses
Anti-B4-bR	B-NHL, CLL, ALL	I	34	350μg/kg	Transaminase elevations (IV) Thrombocytopenia (IV)	19/34 HAMA 19/34 HARA	2 CR, 3 PR, 11 transient responses
Anti-B4-bR	Post-ABMT adjuvant	I	12	280μg/kg	Transaminase elevations (IV) Thrombocytopenia (IV)	5/12 HAMA 7/12 HARA	7 patients in CCR at 31–67 months post-BMT
Anti-B4-bR	Post-ABMT adjuvant	II	49	N/A	N/A	2/49 HAMA 23/49 HARA	27 patients alive in CCR at median of 37 months post-ABMT
Anti-B4-bR	Post-ABMT adjuvant	III	On-going	N/A	N/A	N/A	N/A
Anti-B4-bR	HIV-related B-NHL	I/II	28	140μg/kg[a]	N/A	4/28 HAMA 8/28 HARA	N/A
Anti-B4-bR	HIV-related B-NHL	I	9	Not achieved	Not reached	1/9 HAMA 3/9 HARA	1 CR, 1 PR, 1 mixed response

Table 1. (Cont.)

Immunotoxin	Disease	Phase	Patients (n)	MTD (total dose)	DLT (NCI CTC grade)	HAMA/HARA	Response
Anti-B4-bR	Multiple myeloma	II	5	N/A	Transaminase elevations (IV) Thrombocytopenia (IV) Capillary leak syndrome	1/4 HAMA 2/4 HARA	No clinical responses. One patient in CR at follow-up
Anti-B4-bR	CLL	II	6	N/A	Thrombocytopenia	2/6 HAMA 2/6 HARA	9/14 courses with > 25% decrease in lymphocytes
Anti-My9-bR	AML	I	18	100µg/kg	Capillary leak syndrome Thrombocytopenia	Not available	3 patients with transient decreases in circulating blasts
Anti-CD6-bR	CTCL	I	5	Not reached	Not achieved	3/5 HAMA 3/5 HARA	Not available
N901-bR	Small cell lung cancer	I	21	210µg/kg	Capillary leak syndrome	11/20 HAMA 18/20 HARA	1 PR
N901-bR	Small cell lung cancer (Adjuvant Therapy)	II	9	N/A	Capillary leak syndrome	8/9 HAMA 8/9 HARA	Not available

[a] Anti-B4-bR administered in conjunction with chemotherapy.

administration. Some of these studies were among the first clinical trials of ITs conducted and employed suboptimal dosing schedules and enrolled heavily pretreated patients. These ITs have been used both in vivo for the treatment of patients with relapsed and refractory hematologic malignancies and in vitro for the purging of autologous harvested bone marrow prior to its reinfusion into patients following high dose chemotherapy and radiation therapy.

4.1 Anti-B4-bR

4.1.1 Non-Hodgkin's Lymphoma

Anti-B4-bR is the blocked ricin IT which has been subjected to the most extensive clinical testing. This IT is comprised of blocked ricin and an IgG1 murine MoAb, anti-B4, which binds to the CD19 cell surface antigen (NADLER et al. 1983). CD19 proves to be an exceptionally favorable target for the therapy of B cell neoplasms because it is expressed on malignant B cells in more than 95% of cases of B cell NHL, ALL, and CLL (ANDERSON et al. 1984). The CD19 antigen is expressed throughout B cell ontogeny and represents the earliest detected pan-B cell antigen, enhancing the likelihood that it will be present on the putative clonogenic tumor cell. The antigen is lineage restricted and extensive tissue binding studies fail to identify its expression on other normal tissues. Inasmuch as CD19 is not expressed on hematopoietic stem cells, normal B cells destroyed by the IT can be replenished after therapy.

B cell NHL represents an important disease to target with IT therapy. In fact, NHL is the malignancy which has been treated most frequently with MoAb-based therapies, reflecting both its prevalence and the presence of lineage restricted target antigens. More than 50,000 new cases of NHL are diagnosed each year in the United States with the incidence steadily rising for reasons that are not clear, although a portion of the rising incidence can be attributed to the increased frequency of NHL in patients with HIV infection (PARKER et al. 1996). Approximately 40% of NHL cases are low grade and, while responsive to a wide variety of single agent and combination chemotherapy programs, are nonetheless incurable (ARMITAGE 1993). Of the other 60% of NHL cases, which include intermediate and high grade NHL, only one half can be cured with front-line chemotherapy or bone marrow transplantation.

Cytotoxicity studies were conducted using anti-B4-bR with both the CD19-positive Namalwa cell line and the CD19-negative MOLT-4 cell line (of T cell lineage) (GROSSBARD et al. 1992a). Native ricin demonstrates an IC_{37} value of 4pM against Namalwa cells whereas the IC_{37} value for ricin A-chain alone or conjugated to anti-B4 is 5 logs greater. However, when blocked ricin is conjugated to anti-B4, the IT retains nearly the full potency of native ricin such that the immunoconjugate has an IC_{37} that is only about five-fold higher in concentration than native ricin. When MOLT-4 cells are exposed to anti-B4-bR, the cytotoxicity is 3 logs lower than that seen against the CD19-positive cell line, confirming the antigen-specific cytotoxicity of this IT. Importantly, at concentrations of 1–2nM, which have no effect on MOLT-4 cells, more than 5 logs of Namalwa cells can be killed by anti-B4-bR.

Preclinical in vivo studies of anti-B4-bR in both mice and monkeys were performed to explore potential unanticipated side effects of the IT. Bolus administration of anti-B4-bR produced hepatic toxicity, lymphoid hyperplasia, lethargy, bone marrow hyperplasia, and, at the highest doses, acute tubular necrosis of the kidney and pulmonary alveolar edema. Anti-B4-bR was also administered by continuous IV infusion for 4–7 days in cynomolgus monkeys. Toxicity was diminished with the use of a prolonged infusion with side effects notable for hepatic transaminase elevations, lymphoid and bone marrow hyperplasia, and the absence of capillary leak syndrome. Plateau serum concentrations could be obtained and maintained throughout the treatment period.

The first clinical trial of anti-B4-bR was a phase I study conducted in patients with relapsed B cell neoplasms including NHL, CLL, and ALL (Table 1) (GROSSBARD et al. 1992a). Of the 25 patients treated 23 had B-NHL. Escalating doses of anti-B4-bR ranging from 1µg/kg per day to 60µg/kg per day were administered by daily 1h IV infusion for 5 consecutive days. The MTD was reached at a dose of 50µg/kg per day (total 250µg/kg) with the dose-limiting toxicities (DLTs) defined by transient, reversible grade III elevations of SGOT and SGPT. Other toxicities included fever, hypoalbuminemia, and thrombocytopenia (grade IV). Peak serum levels above 2nM were achieved, and such levels potentially are capable of killing up to 5 logs of malignant B cells in vitro. However, these levels were sustained only transiently thereby inhibiting optimal cytotoxicity. Nine of the 25 patients developed HAMA and/or HARA within 1 month following therapy. One complete response (CR), two partial responses (PRs), and eight transient or mixed responses occurred. This study demonstrated both the safety and biologic activity of anti-B4-bR administration in patients with relapsed B-NHL. However, the study also demonstrated a major shortcoming of bolus injections with this and other ITs, namely, the short-lived peak serum drug concentrations. In vitro studies had demonstrated the dependence of cytotoxicity not only on IT dose, but also on the length of exposure to IT (GROSSBARD et al. 1993b).

Therefore, a second phase I clinical study was initiated which attempted to define the pharmacokinetics, toxicity, and MTD of anti-B4-bR when delivered via prolonged continuous infusion (GROSSBARD et al. 1993b). Thirty-four patients with relapsed B cell neoplasms (26 NHL, 4 CLL, 4 ALL) received escalating doses of anti-B4-bR ranging from 10 to 70µg/kg per day by continuous infusion for 7 days (Table 1). Doses of anti-B4-bR beyond the MTD of 50µg/kg per day for 7 days (total dose 350µg/kg) yielded the DLT of grade IV hepatic transaminase elevations and grade IV thrombocytopenia. Patients treated at or above the dose of 40µg/kg per day achieved serum concentrations capable of killing 4–5 logs of malignant B cells in vitro. Furthermore, these levels could be sustained for up to 96h, which potentially should yield enhanced in vivo cytotoxicity. Of note, lower serum levels were achieved in those patients with CLL and ALL who had a large tumor burden of accessible circulating cells resulting in rapid IT clearance.

While preclinical animal studies suggested that higher doses of anti-B4-bR could be administered by continuous infusion than by bolus injection with lower nonspecific toxicity, this did not prove to be true in humans. Patients receiving continuous infusions did achieve a higher MTD, but at a cost of greater overall side effects as manifested by fevers, nausea, edema, myalgias, hypoalbuminemia, headaches, and capillary leak syndrome. The increased systemic toxicity may be attributable to the prolonged exposure of endothelial cells to IT with subsequent enhanced nonspecific uptake. These added toxicities all were reversible and tolerable. HAMA and/or HARA unfortunately occurred in 24 of the 34 patients although there was some theoretical hope that continuous infusion of anti-B4-bR might decrease the frequency of antibody formation due to the targeting of B cells by the IT. Clinical responses included two CRs, three PRs, and 11 transient responses which indicated biological activity of anti-B4-bR but failed to meet the rigorous criteria for CR or PR. Of note, the two complete responses occurred in those patients on the trial with the lowest tumor burden.

In another phase I clinical trial, McLaughlin et al. (1994) used 28 day continuous infusions of anti-B4-bR to treat patients with B cell neoplasms. At this time, it was appreciated further that anti-B4-bR is a lipophobic compound and dosing was changed to reflect the lean body mass (LBM) of patients rather than their actual weight. The initial cohort of three patients received anti-B4-bR at a dose of 10µg/kg LBM per day for 28 days and subsequent cohorts of patients were treated at doses of 15, 20, and 25 µg/kg LBM per day for 28 days. With this schedule HAMA and HARA occurred in five of 11 evaluable patients, but the median time to HAMA/HARA formation was delayed to 105 days, longer than that seen in earlier studies. Sustained and potentially therapeutic serum levels could be achieved at doses at or above 15µg/kg per day. Two partial responses were achieved in a patient with CLL and a patients with low grade NHL, and three minor responses also were observed. The MTD was not yet reached at a dose of 25µg/kg LBM per day.

Considered together, these phase I studies with anti-B4-bR demonstrated the safety of therapy in patients with relapsed B cell neoplasms. However, they also confirmed that the therapy of bulk disease represents a fundamental difficulty in IT therapy. This finding has been recognized further in a phase II clinical trial using anti-B4-bR administered at doses of 30–50µg/kg per day at 14 day intervals in patients with both relapsed and untreated low grade NHL. One patient, who developed nausea, abdominal pain, and subsequent life-threatening hypotension and thrombocytopenia, died on that trial as a probable complication of severe capillary leak syndrome. No other new toxicities have been observed. Yet even with the inclusion of less heavily pretreated patients at the "optimal" dose of IT, as determined by the earlier studies, relatively few sustained responses have been seen in these patients with bulky NHL. Furthermore, in vitro studies have demonstrated that bulky tumors can exert significant interstitial pressures which limit IT diffusion (Jain and Baxter 1988).

Thus, we planned our next set of clinical investigations to target a population of patients with minimal tumor burdens. Patients undergoing high dose myeloablative therapy followed by ABMT for the treatment of chemosensitive relapsed NHL achieve high rates of CR early after therapy. However, 55%–85% of these patients will relapse within 24 months due to chemoresistant tumor cells harbored within the patient or occult tumor cells reinfused with the autologous marrow (PHILIP et al. 1995; FREEMAN and NADLER 1993). This group of patients should have a negligible tumor burden immediately after ABMT and should prove to be an optimal group to treat with anti-B4-bR as an adjuvant therapy. In addition, because of the unique cytotoxic mechanism of this IT, the potential exists to kill residual tumor cells which are resistant to the high dose therapy.

In a phase I trial, 12 patients in CR after ABMT for B-NHL received escalating doses of anti-B4-bR, from 20–50µg/kg per day for 7 days by continuous infusion (GROSSBARD et al. 1993a). As in the earlier studies, the DLTs were grade IV transaminase elevations and thrombocytopenia. It is important to recognize that these patients began therapy with low platelet counts inasmuch as they received therapy soon after engraftment of bone marrow post-ABMT. Some manifestations of capillary leak syndrome also were observed, but these were not dose-limiting. The MTD of 40µg/kg per day for 7 days (total dose 280µg/kg) was lower in this trial than in the previous investigations which was not surprising since these patients had negligible tumor burdens. Although patients are profoundly immunosuppressed following ABMT, seven patients still developed HAMA and/or HARA attesting to the immunogenicity of this IT. With median follow-up of more than 4 years post-ABMT, seven patients remain in CR.

A subsequent phase II trial of anti-B4-bR adjuvant therapy post-ABMT also has been completed (GROSSBARD et al. 1994). In this trial, the dose and schedule of anti-B4-bR administration were altered. Whereas HAMA and HARA detection typically occurs no sooner than 3 weeks following therapy with anti-B4-bR, the toxic effects of the IT usually resolve significantly within 7 days of completing therapy. Thus, in the phase II trial, patients were eligible for retreatment at 14 day intervals rather than the 28 day intervals used in the earlier trial. In addition, the administered dose was lowered to 30µg/kg per day for 7 days in an attempt to lower toxicity while still achieving potentially therapeutic serum levels. Finally, patients on this trial were dosed according to their LBM.

Forty-nine patients were treated at a mean of 105 days post-ABMT. Thirty-four patients received two or more courses of therapy, demonstrating that patients could be retreated safely using this schedule. HAMA and/or HARA eventually occurred in 23 patients at a median of 22 days post-initiation of therapy. Toxicity was markedly decreased as compared with the phase I adjuvant trial, with only three patients developing grade IV thrombocytopenia. There were no cases of grade IV hepatotoxicity and only two patients had grade III transaminase elevations. To date 19 patients have relapsed, 27 are alive and in CR (at a median of 37 months post-ABMT), and three have died in CR.

Although the phase I and II trials of anti-B4-bR post-ABMT provided intriguing data regarding the safety and pharmacokinetics of administering anti-B4-bR in this setting, they offered no definitive data on the efficacy of this approach. A phase III trial being conducted under the auspices of the Cancer and Leukemia

Group B is designed to address the question of efficacy. Patients with B-NHL who are in CR 60–120 days after ABMT are randomized to receive no further therapy or two courses of anti-B4-bR therapy at 30µg/kg for LBM per day by 7 day continuous infusion. To date, more than 350 patients have been registered for the ABMT phase of this trial and 120 patients have been randomized to receive either IT therapy or no further therapy. This is the first phase III trial to address the in vivo clinical efficacy of any IT. The study should complete accrual in 1997 and preliminary results may be available shortly thereafter.

A similar phase II adjuvant trial using anti-B4-bR was conducted in patients with NHL and minimal residual disease following conventional chemotherapy with Pro-MACE-CytaBOM, an aggressive third generation chemotherapy regimen with high response rates in untreated NHL (Longo, personal communication). After receiving six to eight cycles of chemotherapy, 37 patients with advanced indolent NHL received anti-B4-bR at a dose of 30µg/kg for LBM per day. Patients received up to six cycles of anti-B4-bR therapy given at 14 day intervals. Analysis of the results of this trial are in progress. The investigators are using the *bcl*-2 proto-oncogene as a surrogate marker of tumor cells in patients with low grade NHL. This translocation is present in 85% of patients with low grade B-NHL (YUNIS et al. 1982; WEISS et al. 1987).

Anti-B4-bR also has been used in vitro to purge the harvested bone marrows of patients with NHL prior to reinfusion during ABMT. Because bone marrow obtained from patients in apparent clinical CR from NHL still can harbor residual lymphoma cells, there are theoretical advantages to cleansing the marrow. One approach previously employed has been to incubate the marrow together with MoAbs (targeting antigens on the surface of leukemic cells) and complement. However, complement is expensive and different lots of complement have varying activity. ITs potentially provide an effective cytotoxic agent for incubation with marrow with predictable potential to deplete malignant cells. The potential of anti-B4-bR to eradicate residual CD19-positive tumor cells from marrow has been described (ROY et al. 1995b). Anti-B4-bR in concentrations > 5nM incubated with marrow for 5h could eliminate more than 3 logs of either Nalm-6 or Namalwa cells (CD19-positive cell lines) added to the marrow sample. This system was designed to mimic the clinical scenario of 5% marrow involvement by residual lymphoma cells following a bone marrow harvest. Anti-B4-bR showed little effect on normal hematopoietic precursors.

In a subsequent clinical trial, anti-B4-bR was used to purge bone marrows obtained from 41 patients with NHL and poor prognostic features including the failure to achieve CR after conventional therapy (ROY et al. 1995a). Median age at ABMT was 44 years with 15 female and 26 male patients. Marrow was incubated with anti-B4-bR at a concentration of 5nM. Minimal effect was seen on hematopoietic precursors (CFU-GM, CFU-E, BFU-E). Stable engraftment of marrow occurred in all patients with a median time to > 500 granulocytes of 21 days and a median time to > 20,000 platelets of 26 days. The Kaplan-Meier 3 year overall survival was 77% and the disease-free survival was 62%.

Several other areas of clinical investigation also are being explored with the anti-B4-bR IT. The treatment of AIDS-related NHL presents particular challenges with the use of traditional cytotoxic therapies because of the poor tolerance these patients have for myelosuppression and the further insult that cytotoxic chemotherapy adds to their immune systems. As supportive care improves and patients with AIDS live for longer durations, the risk of developing NHL increases. As many as 30%–40% of AIDS patients ultimately may develop NHL if they survive long enough (PLUDA et al. 1990). Even the most successful combination chemotherapy regimens have achieved only 50% CR rates with a median survival of 5.6 months (LEVINE et al. 1991; KAPLAN et al. 1995). Anti-B4-bR offers a non-myelosuppressive therapy for these patients with specific cytotoxicity.

An initial phase I study demonstrated the biological activity of anti-B4-bR in AIDS patients with NHL (TULPULE et al. 1994). Patients with relapsed AIDS-related NHL received escalating doses of anti-B4-bR administered by 28 day continuous infusion. In the first nine patients treated, one CR and one PR were observed. A second phase I/II trial used anti-B4-bR in conjunction with m-BACOD (methotrexate, bleomycin, doxorubicin, cyclophosphamide, vincristine, and dexamethasone) chemotherapy to treat patients with newly diagnosed AIDS-related NHL (SCADDEN et al. 1993; FRANKEL et al. 1996). Patients received two cycles of chemotherapy, and if responding to therapy, anti-B4-bR by 7 day continuous infusion (20µg/kg per day) in conjunction with the third and fourth cycles of therapy. Toxicities included grade III fever, myalgias, nausea, vomiting, and fatigue. These highly immunocompromised patients were able to mount an immune response to the IT with eight of 28 patients developing HAMA/HARA. However, antibodies developed at a median of 48 days post-therapy, a longer time interval than that observed in previous studies with anti-B4-bR in non-AIDS patients.

In a recently completed trial, patients with AIDS-related NHL were treated with standard dose CHOP therapy for up to eight cycles. With the third and fifth cycles, responding patients received a 28 day continuous infusion of anti-B4-bR. Safety and toxicity data from this latter trial still are under analysis and may be used to form the basis of a randomized trial in AIDS-related NHL of CHOP vs CHOP + anti-B4-bR.

Finally, preclinical studies have established potential synergistic cytotoxicity of anti-B4-bR with conventional chemotherapeutic agents (O'CONNOR et al. 1995; LIU et al. 1996). For example, anti-B4-bR has been used in combination with cyclophosphamide, vincristine, etoposide and doxorubicin to treat SCID mice bearing Namalwa tumors. Either combination chemotherapy or anti-B4-bR alone offers some cytotoxicity, with an enhanced life span of tumor-bearing mice as compared with untreated controls. However, with the use of both combination chemotherapy and anti-B4-bR there is synergistic cytotoxicity with 20% of mice apparently cured of their lymphoma. These studies form the basis of an on-going clinical trial of anti-B4-bR in combination with these chemotherapy agents.

4.1.2 Chronic Lymphocytic Leukemia and Acute Lymphoblastic Leukemia

Limited experience also has been accrued with this IT for the treatment of patients with both CLL and ALL. The data acquired from the few leukemia patients enrolled in the original phase I studies of anti-B4-bR in patients with leukemia demonstrated a significant difference in the pharmacokinetic profile of this agent in patients with large numbers of circulating tumor cells (GROSSBARD et al. 1993b). Peak serum levels of IT in patients with CLL and ALL were dramatically lower than those in patients with NHL, indicating high clearance rates of IT from serum. Side effects of therapy in these patients were negligible, reflecting the rapid clearance of the IT. Only transient reductions of circulating malignant cells were observed, and there was no significant effect on bone marrow involvement.

Subsequently, a phase II study was undertaken in patients with CLL (GROSSBARD et al. 1995). Six patients with refractory CLL received anti-B4-bR at a dose of 30µg/kg per day for 7 days or 50µg/kg per day for 7 days by continuous infusion. Patients were eligible for retreatment at 14 day intervals. A total of 14 courses of therapy were administered, and decreases of 25% or greater in circulating lymphocytes were observed in nine courses. As in the phase I studies, peak serum levels of IT (0.14nM) were below those deemed to be potentially therapeutic. Two of six patients developed HAMA/HARA. Toxicities included grade IV thrombocytopenia (two patients), grade II fever and rigors (one patient), and grade III anemia (one patient).

SZATROWSKI et al. (1995) reported the preliminary results of a phase II trial using anti-B4-bR as part of the consolidation therapy for adult patients with B-ALL. Forty-six patients whose ALL cells were CD19-positive and who remained in CR after one course of consolidation therapy received anti-B4-bR at a dose of 30µg/kg LBM per day for up to two 7 day continuous infusions at 14 day intervals. Toxicity was notable for transaminase elevations, lymphopenia, and flu-like symptoms. Two patients experienced chest pain accompanied by the development of pleural effusions. With a median follow-up of 9.6 months, the median duration of CR for patients treated with anti-B4-bR was 10.2 months. The median duration of CR for patients receiving a similar ALL treatment program without anti-B4-bR was 9.7 months. The results of molecular studies to monitor the efficacy of anti-B4-bR therapy in eradicating minimal residual disease on this study are pending.

4.1.3 Multiple Myeloma

Multiple myeloma (MM) is a plasma cell neoplasm, with approximately 14,000 new cases diagnosed each year in the United States (PARKER et al. 1996). The median survival of patients is 36 months. Despite the use of aggressive combination chemotherapy, adjuvant therapy with interferon-α and bone marrow transplantation, the outcome has not been altered convincingly (SALMON and CASSADY 1993). Although the CD19 antigen is not expressed on normal or malignant plasma cells, it is likely to be expressed on the clonogenic myeloma tumor cell because it appears so early in B cell ontogeny. Evidence suggests that the self-renewal capacity of the malignant cell in myeloma lies in a "pre-myeloma" compartment with cells having the morphologic and immunophenotypic features of lymphocytes (BILLADEAU et al. 1993). Hence, treatment of MM with anti-B4-bR may provide cytotoxicity to the malignant stem cell while circumventing rapid clearance of the IT by an excess of CD19-positive tumor cells.

Five patients with relapsed and refractory MM were treated with a 7 day continuous infusion of anti-B4-bR on a phase II trial (Grossbard et al. 1995). Although the initial protocol was designed to treat patients at a dose of 40µg/kg per day for 7 days (the same dose used in the low tumor burden adjuvant NHL setting), this dose proved to have intolerable toxicity in two of the first four patients treated. Thus, the dose was lowered to 30µg/kg per day for 7 days in the fifth patient. Exceptionally high serum IT levels were achieved in the two patients exhibiting intolerable toxicity, with peak levels (that did not plateau) in excess of 2.7nM. Such levels were much higher than those seen when comparable IT doses were used to treat patients with NHL. Possibly, these altered pharmacokinetics reflect reduced nonspecific uptake of anti-B4-bR by the reticuloendothelial system in patients with a circulating paraprotein. However, one of these two patients had a nonsecretory myeloma. The other three patients had IT serum levels (1–2nM) comparable to those described for NHL patients treated at similar doses of IT. Toxicity was not qualitatively different from that seen in previous clinical trials using anti-B4-bR, but it was more severe. Three patients had declines in performance status during therapy, and two patients had grade IV thrombocytopenia. One patient died following anti-B4-bR therapy, secondary to neurologic toxicity and akinetic mutism. This side effect was likely due to progressive MM and hypercalcemia, although a contribution of anti-B4-bR in the patient's demise cannot be excluded. No reductions in paraprotein were observed within 28 days of anti-B4-bR therapy, but such reductions may not be expected within this interval since circulating paraprotein and antigen-negative plasma cells have a long circulatory half-life. One patient with a nonsecretory myeloma remains in CR more than 3 years out from the completion of therapy. In light of the toxicity and possible altered pharmacokinetics in patients with MM, the clinical trial was closed early. A traditional phase I trial will be required in this disease to define appropriate doses and schedules of anti-B4-bR administration.

4.2 Anti-My9-bR

A second IT also has been developed for the treatment of patients with hematologic malignancies. Anti-My9-bR is an immunoconjugate between the anti-My9 (CD33) antibody and blocked ricin. The anti-My9 MoAb identifies a myeloid lineage restricted surface antigen which appears in myeloid development at the level of the CFU-GEMM, a colony forming cell capable of giving rise to granulocytes, erythrocytes, monocytes, and megakaryocytes. This antigen is expressed on leukemic cells in more than 80% of cases of AML and also on more than 80% of cases of chronic myelogenous leukemia (CML) in blast crisis (Griffin et al. 1984). AML is the most common acute leukemia of adults. While 50%–80% of patients can enter remission using standard induction chemotherapy regimens, fewer than 30% of these patients are cured with this initial therapy.

The in vitro specificity and cytotoxicity of the IT was examined on normal and leukemic myeloid and nonmyeloid cells (Roy et al. 1991). When cells from the My9 antigen-positive myeloid leukemia cell line HL-60 were exposed to 10^{-8}M concentrations of anti-My9-bR for 2h, 4–5 logs of cells could be killed. Blocked ricin alone required more than 1000 times the dose to achieve similar cytotoxicity. If a 100-fold excess of anti-My9 antibody is added to the assay system, cytotoxicity for HL-60 cells is blocked completely. This IT has relatively little toxicity for normal hematopoietic progenitor cells, with less than 1 log kill of CFU-GEMM and CFU-E and 1–2 logs kill of BFU-E at concentrations of anti-My9-bR comparable to those which are cytotoxic for HL-60 cells.

Preclinical studies were designed to examine the cross-reactivity of the anti-My9 MoAb with nonhematopoietic tissues (unpublished data). Scattered antigen-positive macrophages were identified in spleen, lung, liver and the interstitium of the testes. No epithelial or endothelial staining was identified, but there was minor staining of sweat ducts, salivary gland ducts, and goblet cells in the gastrointestinal tract. Murine and monkey toxicity studies demonstrated that bolus infusions of anti-My9-bR resulted in periportal inflammation, hepatic necrosis at the highest doses, bone marrow hyperplasia, lymphoid hyperplasia, and acute tubular necrosis. Similar changes were seen using continuous infusions of the IT in cynomolgus monkeys.

A phase I trial was conducted using anti-My9-bR to treat patients with relapsed AML and CML in myeloid blast crisis whose leukemic cells expressed the CD33 antigen (Grossbard et al., unpublished data). Patients in the initial five cohorts received bolus doses of IT ranging from 2 to 32µg/kg followed by a 5 day continuous infusion at 12.5–200µg/kg total dose. Eighteen patients were treated on the trial and patients in the first four cohorts experienced mild side effects including headaches, mild hypotension, nausea, and fever. One patient had mild elevations of hepatic transaminases. No evidence of efficacy was observed in these patients. Patients in the fifth cohort, who received a bolus dose of 32µg/kg followed by a 5 day infusion of 200µg/kg total dose (40µg/kg per day), experienced increased toxicity, including a patient who died on day 9 of the protocol due to complications of capillary leak syndrome and respiratory distress.

Because of this severe toxicity, the bolus dose at initiation of therapy was eliminated since it was felt to contribute to toxicity without enhancing efficacy. Thus, the next cohort of patients was treated at a dose of 20µg/kg per day for 5 days, the dose level below that at which lethal toxicity occurred. The three patients at this dose level experienced side effects including fever, edema, hypoalbuminemia, nausea, and diarrhea, but had no grade III or IV toxicity. The next cohort of patients was treated at a dose of 30µg/kg per day for 5 days. The first patient tolerated therapy well, without major side effects, but the second patient developed severe capillary leak syndrome with hypoalbuminemia, edema, and respiratory failure and died secondary to IT toxicity. The severe toxicity on this trial which appeared at dose levels below those which could saturate tumor antigen binding sites and provide therapeutic serum levels led to termination of the study.

Nevertheless, the potent in vitro cytotoxicity of this IT for leukemic cells bearing the My9 antigen still could be exploited by using the IT for purging of leukemic cells from bone marrow harvests prior to reinfusing these cells in patients undergoing ABMT (Roy et al. 1991). ABMT is an important therapeutic option for patients with relapsed AML who lack an allogeneic marrow donor. In this setting, the systemic toxicity of anti-My9-bR is not a concern and sufficiently cytotoxic doses can be delivered to deplete residual leukemic cells while preserving progenitor cell capability (La Russa et al. 1992).

In an initial clinical trial, 15 patients with AML either in first remission (6 patients) or second remission (9 patients) received autologous marrow treated with anti-My9-bR after myeloablative therapy with busulfan and cyclophosphamide (Roy et al. 1993). Although anti-My9-bR depleted 48% of BFU-E and more than 75% of CFU-GM, all patients demonstrated stable engraftment with a median time to > 500 granulocytes of 37 days and to > 20,000 platelets of 60 days. In fact, anti-My9-bR depleted fewer CFU-GM from marrow than treatment with anti-My9 MoAb plus complement (Robertson et al. 1993). The estimated overall survival at 2 years was 66% and the estimated disease-free survival was 42%.

4.3 Anti-CD6-bR

Cutaneous T cell lymphoma (CTCL) is an often indolent, but occasionally aggressive, malignancy which presents with skin manifestations including eczema and erythema (Bunn and Hoppe 1993). The disease is uncommon, with approximately 600 new cases diagnosed each year in the United States. Because CTCL often presents with well vascularized plaques of skin disease, it should be a suitable malignancy for IT therapy, since bulky masses may not exist to impair IT delivery.

Anti-CD6-bR links blocked ricin with an anti-CD6 MoAb (Collinson et al. 1994). The resultant IT targets cells containing the CD6 antigen which is expressed on more than 80% of mature T cells. When the IT is used to target MOLT-4 cells, a CD6 bearing cell line, the IC_{37} is 4pM. Nonspecific toxicity for the B cell line Namalwa is more than 750-fold lower. The systemic toxicity of this agent in preclinical animal studies was similar to that observed with anti-B4-bR. A phase I dose escalation trial using this IT in patients with relapsed or refractory CTCL has been initiated.

5 Blocked Ricin Immunotoxin Therapy of Solid Tumors: N901-bR

The application of IT therapy to solid tumors has lagged behind that in hematologic malignancies (Grossbard and Nadler 1992). Two factors contribute significantly to this delay. First, it has been difficult to identify tumor-specific antigens on solid tumors. Indeed, the coexpression of many of the appropriate antigen targets on normal tissues precludes the safe use of most antibodies for IT therapy.

For example, ITs constructed to target breast cancer and ovarian cancer were administered to patients and led to devastating neurologic toxicity due to unanticipated binding of the antibody to neural tissues secondary to antigen coexpression (GOULD et al. 1989; PAI et al. 1991). Second, solid tumors often present as large bulky masses making tumor penetration difficult and leading to relative antigen inaccessibility.

N901-bR is an IT which has been constructed for the treatment of SCLC. The N901 antibody is an IgG1 murine MoAb which binds to the CD56 (NKH-1) surface antigen which is expressed by normal natural killer cells (GRIFFIN et al. 1983). In addition, the antigen is present on nearly all SCLC cell lines and fresh human tumor tissue that have been tested. N901-bR demonstrates high cytotoxicity in vitro for CD56-positive SW-2 cells, a cell line derived from SCLC. The IC_{37} for this cell line after exposure to N901-bR for 24h is 14.5pM, more than 700-fold lower than the IC_{37} for Namalwa cells (which do not express the target antigen). Extended exposure times yield progressively lower IC_{37} values, indicating that the cytotoxicity of N901-bR is a function of both concentration and exposure time.

Screening of nonhuman primate tissues as well as human tissues obtained from tissue banks revealed that N901-bR bound to the majority of cells of neuroectodermal origin, including astrocytes and neurons in the central nervous system, neuroendocrine cells in the pancreas and adrenal cortex, and peripheral nerves (LYNCH et al., unpublished data). In addition, N901-bR bound to cardiac muscle. Preclinical murine and monkey studies demonstrated toxicities including hepatic transaminase elevations, chronic lung inflammation, bile duct hyperplasia, myocardial cell necrosis, and subacute to chronic myocardial inflammation. Additional monkey studies were designed specifically to assess potential neurotoxicity of N901-bR. Doses of 505 or 1010μg/kg given by 6 day continuous infusion caused mild abnormalities of motor conduction as evidenced by electromyogram abnormalities. None of the monkeys demonstrated clinical manifestations of neurotoxicity.

With preclinical testing completed, an initial phase I trial of N901-bR was conducted in 21 patients with relapsed or refractory SCLC (Table 1) (LYNCH et al. 1995). Cohorts of three patients were treated at doses ranging from 5 to 40μg/kg per day by 7 day continuous infusion. At the first three dose levels, the day one dose was administered as a bolus infusion over 60 min to permit an assessment of bolus pharmacokinetics. The initial 13 patients were dosed by actual body weight, while the last eight patients were dosed by calculated lean body weight. As was true for anti-B4-bR, the peak concentration of N901-bR was achieved approximately 1h after the bolus injection and then declined to less than one half the peak concentration over the next 5h. When continuous infusions of N901-bR were administered, a plateau concentration could be achieved at approximately day 4 and be maintained until day 7. Serum concentrations in the range of 90ng/ml were achieved, and such concentrations can kill more than 4 logs of N901 antigen-positive cells in vitro with 24h exposure to the IT. In three patients, tissue samples were obtained during treatment to investigate whether the IT reached the targeted tissue. By immunoperoxidase staining, N901-bR could be identified binding to tumor cells in all instances.

The DLT of N901-bR was capillary leak syndrome, characterized by hypoalbuminemia, hypotension, peripheral edema, and dyspnea. Two patients at the MTD of 40μg/kg per day for 7 days developed hypotension requiring hospitalization for greater than 48h, and one patient required an infusion of dopamine to maintain a systolic blood pressure above 90mm Hg. To monitor potential cardiac toxicity, all patients received Holter monitoring during the first 48h of therapy. Fourteen patients developed sinus tachycardia during the infusion, likely secondary to hypovolemia which occurred as a manifestation of capillary leak syndrome. One patient developed atrial fibrillation which did not necessitate discontinuation of the infusion. In 15 of 16 patients, there was no change in the left ventricular ejection fraction following therapy. One patient had a myocardial infarction on day 8 of therapy as detected by a routine electrocardiogram showing an acute anterior wall myocardial infarction. Of note, this patient had prior coronary artery disease, diabetes, hypertension, and mediastinal radiation. It is impossible to determine whether N901-bR contributed to this ischemic cardiac event. Two of the other 16 patients who were monitored also showed an increase in CPK with therapy, and one of these patients had a mild decline in left ventricular ejection fraction from 66% to 56% post-therapy.

Neurologic toxicity also was examined closely in patients treated on this trial. Because most patients had received prior cis-platinum therapy for their disease, 11 patients had a mild to moderate baseline peripheral neuropathy. In addition, four patients had evidence of Horner's syndrome. Baseline focal peripheral neuropathies, radicular signs, and cerebellar ataxia also were observed. Neurophysiological studies done pre- and post-therapy indicated a decline in amplitude for all sensory and motor nerves tested. Nevertheless, no patient developed any clinically significant neurological signs or symptoms following N901-bR therapy.

Twenty of the patients were evaluated for HAMA and HARA. In contrast to patients with NHL, patients with SCLC have less baseline immune system impairment and, not surprisingly, develop anti-mouse and anti-ricin antibodies at a high frequency. Seventeen patients had evidence of HARA and 11 patients had evidence of HAMA within 28 days after initiating therapy. An additional patient developed HARA at day 34. This high rate of antibody formation precluded the delivery of repeat courses of therapy to patients.

Six of the patients had stable disease 1 month following treatment, while an additional 14 patients showed evidence of progression. One patient treated at 30μg/kg per day for 7 days had a PR with resolution of right upper lobe and left lower lobe CT scan abnormalities and a 50% reduction in size of a right lower lobe mass. The PR persisted for 3 months without additional therapy.

In sum, this phase I clinical trial indicated that N901-bR could be administered to patients with relapsed SCLC with tolerable and reversible toxicities. The DLT of capillary leak syndrome is commonly seen with ITs. Although there was evidence of binding of N901-bR to tumor, it is unclear whether all sites of bulky disease are exposed to therapeutic concentrations of N901-bR. The high frequency of antibody formation also is limiting. It is difficult to imagine that a single infusion of IT will kill enough tumor cells to effect a clinical PR or CR in many patients.

As with anti-B4-bR, N901-bR can be employed in the adjuvant setting following the completion of induction chemotherapy. For patients with extensive stage SCLC, conventional chemotherapy regimens are capable of inducing remissions in approximately 60% of patients. However, no patients are cured and the median survival is in the range of 9 months. While only 5%–10% of patients with limited stage SCLC may be cured of their disease, these patients nevertheless have extraordinarily high remission rates after initial chemotherapy with or without radiation therapy. Hence, SCLC is an optimal disease in which to assess the efficacy of adjuvant IT therapy.

A phase II trial using N901-bR to treat patients with reduced tumor burdens following induction therapy has been initiated (LYNCH et al. 1995). Eligible patients are in CR or near CR within 60 days of receiving their final chemotherapy or radiation therapy. All patients receive a 7 day continuous infusion of N901-bR at a dose of 30µg/kg LBM per day for 7 days. By treating patients with negligible tumor burdens, the obstacles of tumor bulk and HAMA/HARA formation may be circumvented. Perhaps a single cycle of therapy in these patients can effect enough cytotoxicity to enhance the remission duration and cure rates. To date, nine patients have been treated on this protocol. No new toxicities have been seen as compared with the initial study. Capillary leak syndrome has occurred frequently, and one patient died secondary to respiratory failure and hypotension likely secondary to capillary leak syndrome. At autopsy, the patient was found to have residual SCLC. Whether N901-bR will have acceptable toxicity and efficacy in the adjuvant setting remains to be determined.

6 Conclusions

Four bR-ITs now have been used in human clinical trials. These ITs have been used to treat patients with both hematologic malignancies and solid tumors. From these trials, several conclusions already can be made:

First, the similarity between these ITs in terms of their in vivo toxicity is striking. Despite the use of different antibodies and target antigens, all of these agents cause capillary leak syndrome, transient liver enzyme elevations, and thrombocytopenia as side effects. Hence, the antibodies to which these toxins are conjugated confer the necessary specificity to the blocked ricin toxin and the few side effects of therapy that may be antibody mediated do not appear to be dose-limiting.

Second, all of these agents have been demonstrated to have biologic activity, even in pretreated patients with bulky relapsed disease. In each instance, limitations exist to the efficacy of therapy in patients with bulky tumors, and future clinical efforts will best be directed toward the testing of these agents in the minimal residual disease state. Preliminary studies with both anti-B4-bR and N901-bR demonstrate that adjuvant therapy can be accomplished safely with these agents.

Third, these compounds are immunogenic, minimizing the potential to deliver repeat courses of therapy. However, in the case of anti-B4-bR, it may be possible to develop alternative infusion schedules (e.g., 28 day continuous infusion) which suppress B cells and limit the ability to mount an immune response. Similarly, when anti-B4-bR has been used in conjunction with ProMACE-CytaBOM chemotherapy, multiple cycles of the IT can be delivered. Continued efforts must be directed at developing alternative infusion schedules, humanizing the antibodies, producing a recombinant toxin, or suppressing the patient's immune system in order to circumvent the obstacle of HAMA/HARA formation.

Valuable lessons have been learned from the first generation of clinical studies with each of the ITs detailed in this chapter. Within the next few years, pivotal studies will have been completed for one or more of these agents that will better define their efficacy and their role in cancer therapy.

References

Anderson KC, Slaughenhoupt B, Bates MP, Pinkus G, Schlossman SF, Nadler LM (1984) Expression of human B cell associated antigens on leukemias and lymphomas. Blood 63:1424–1433

Armitage JO (1993) Treatment of non-Hodgkin's lymphoma. N Engl J Med 328:1023–1030

Billadeau D, Ahmann G, Greipp G, Van Ness B (1993) The bone marrow of multiple myeloma patients contains B cell populations at different stages of differentiation that are clonally related to the malignant plasma cell. J Exp Med 178:1023–1031

Blakey DC, Watson GJ, Knowles PP, Thorpe PE (1987) Effect of chemical deglycosylation of ricin A chain on the in vivo fate and cytotoxic activity of an immunotoxin composed of ricin A-chain and anti-Thy 1.1 antibody. Cancer Res 47:947–952

Bunn PA Jr, Hoppe RT (1993) Cutaneous lymphomas. In: Devita VT Jr, Hellman S, Rosenberg SA (eds) Cancer: principles and practice of oncology, fourth edition. Lippincott, Philadelphia

Collinson AR, Lambert JM, Liu Y, O'Dea C, Shah SA, Rasmussen RA, Goldmacher VS (1994) anti-CD6-blocked ricin: an anti-pan T-cell immunotoxin. Int J Immunopharmacol 16:37–49

Endo Y, Mitsui K, Motizuki M, Tsurugi K (1987) The mechanism of action of ricin and related toxic lectins on eukaryotic ribosomes. J Biol Chem 262:5908–5912

Fodstad O, Kvalheim G, Godal A, Lotsberg J, Aamdal S, Host H, Pihl A (1984) Phase I study of the plant protein ricin. Cancer Res 44:862–865

Frankel AE, FitzGerald D, Siegall C, Press OW (1996) Advances in immunotoxin biology and therapy: asummary of the 4th international symposium on immunotoxins. Cancer Res 56:926–932

Freedman AS, Nadler LM (1993) Which patients with relapsed non-Hodgkin's lymphoma benefit from high-dose therapy and hematopoietic stem-cell transplantation? J Clin Oncol 11:1841–1843

Goldmacher VS, Lambert JM, Blattler WA (1992) The specific cytotoxicity of immunoconjugates containing blocked ricin is dependent on the residual binding capacity of blocked ricin: evidence that the membrane binding and A-chain translocation activities of ricin cannot be separated. Biochem Biophys Res Commun 183:758–766

Gould BJ, Borowitz MJ, Groves ES, Carter PW, Anthony D, Weiner LM, Frankel AE (1989) Phase I study of an anti-breast cancer immunotoxin by continuous infusion: report of a targeted toxic effect not predicted by animal studies. J Natl Cancer Inst 81:775–781

Griffin JD, Hercend T, Beveridge RP, Schlossman SF (1983) Characterization of an antigen expressed by human natural killer cells. J Immunol 130:2947–2951

Griffin JD, Linch D, Sabbath K, Larcom P, Schlossman SF (1984) A monoclonal antibody reactive with normal and leukemic progenitor cells. Leuk Res 8:521–534

Grossbard ML, Nadler LM (1992) Immunotoxin therapy of malignancy. In: Devita VT Jr, Hellman S, Rosenberg SA (eds) Important advances in oncology 1992. Lippincott, Philadelphia

Grossbard ML, Freedman AS, Ritz J, Coral F, Goldmacher VS, Eliseo L, Spector N, Dear K, Lambert JM, Blattler WA, Taylor JA, Nadler LM (1992a) Serotherapy of B cell neoplasms with anti-B4-blocked ricin. Blood 79:576–585

Grossbard ML, Lambert JM, Goldmacher VS, Blattler WA, Nadler LM (1992b) Correlation between in vivo toxicity and preclinical in vitro parameters for the immunotoxin anti-B4-blocked ricin. Cancer Res 52:4200–4207

Grossbard ML, Press OW, Appelbaum FR, Bernstein ID, Nadler LM (1992c) Monoclonal antibody-based therapies of leukemia and lymphoma. Blood 80:863–878

Grossbard ML, Gribben JG, Freedman AS, Lambert JM, Kinsella J, Rabinowe SN, Eliseo L, Taylor JA, Blattler WA, Epstein CL, Nadler LM (1993a) Adjuvant immunotoxin therapy with anti-B4-blocked ricin after autologous bone marrow transplantation for patients with B cell non-Hodgkin's lymphoma. Blood 81:2262–2271

Grossbard ML, Lambert JM, Goldmacher VS, Spector NL, Kinsella J, Eliseo L, Coral F, Taylor JA, Blattler WA, Epstein CL, Nadler LM (1993b) anti-B4-blocked ricin: a phase I trial of 7-day continuous infusion in patients with B cell neoplasms. J Clin Oncol 11:726–737

Grossbard ML, O'Day S, Gribben JG, Kolesar C, Freedman AS, Rabinowe SN, Neuberg D, Esseltine DL, Epstein CL, Nadler LM (1994) A phase II study of anti-B4-blocked ricin therapy following autologous bone marrow transplantation (ABMT) for B cell non-Hodgkin's lymphoma. Proc Am Soc Clin Oncol 13:293

Grossbard ML, Fidias P, Bernstein ZP, Vose J, Schuster M, Foon KA, Esseltine DL, Anderson KC, Nadler LM (1995) Phase II studies of anti-B4-blocked ricin (Anti-B4-bR) in multiple myeloma (MM) and chronic lymphocytic leukemia (CLL). Proc ASCO 14:422

Jain RK, Baxter LT (1988) Mechanisms of heterogeneous distribution of monoclonal antibodies and other macromolecules in tumors: significance of elevated interstitial pressure. Cancer Res 48:7022–7032

Kaplan L, Straus D, Testa M, Levine AM (1995) Randomized trial of standard dose mBACOD with GM-CSF vs reduced dose mBACOD for systemic HIV-associated lymphoma. Proc Am Soc Clin Oncol 14:288

Lambert JM, Goldmacher VS, Collinson AR, Nadler LM, Blattler WA (1991a) An immunotoxin prepared with blocked ricin: a natural plant toxin adapted for therapeutic use. Cancer Res 51:6236–6242

Lambert JM, McIntyre G, Gauthier MN, Zullo D, Rao V, Steeves RM, Goldmacher VS, Blattler WA (1991b) The galactose-binding sites of the cytotoxic lectin ricin can be chemically blocked in high yield with reactive ligands prepared by chemical modification of glycopeptides containing triantennary N-linked oligosaccharides. Biochemistry 30:3234–3247

La Russa VF, Griffin JD, Kessler SW, Cutting MA, Knight RD, Blattler WA, Lambert JM, Wright DG (1992) Effects of anti-CD33 blocked ricin immunotoxin on the capacity of CD34+ human marrow cells to establish in vitro hematopoiesis in long-term marrow cultures. Exp Hematol 20:442–448

LeMaistre CF, Rosen S, Frankel A, Kornfeld S, Saria E, Meneghetti C, Drasjek J, Fishwild D, Scannon P, Byers V (1991) Phase I trial of H65-RTA immunoconjugate in patients with T-cell lymphoma. Blood 78:1173–1182

Levine AM, Wernz JC, Kaplan L, Rodman N, Cohen P, Metroka C, Bennett JM, Rarick MU, Walsh C, Kahn J, Miles S, Ehmann WC, Feinberg J, Nathwani B, Gill PS, Mitsuyasu R (1991) Low-dose chemotherapy with central nervous system prophylaxis and zidovudine maintenance in AIDS-related lymphoma. JAMA 266:84–88

Liu C, Lambert JM, Teicher BA, Blattler WA, O'Connor R (1996) Cure of multidrug-resistant human B cell lymphoma xenografts by combinations of anti-B4-blocked ricin and chemotherapeutic drugs. Blood 87:3892–3898

Lynch TJ, Grossbard M, Fidias P, Bartholomay M, Coral F, Salgia R, Elias AD, Skarin A, Sheffner J, Wen P, Arinello P, Bramen G, Esseltine D, Ritz J (1995) Immunotoxin therapy of small cell lung cancer (SCLC): clinical trials of N901-blocked ricin (N901-bR). Proc Am Soc Clin Oncol 14:424

McLaughlin P, Murray JL, Rosenblum M, Brewer H, LeBherz D, O'Brien S, Hagemeister FB, Epstein C, Esseltine D, Keating M (1994) Phase I trial of anti-B4-blocked ricin (B4bR) by 28-day continuous infusion (CI). Proc AACR 35:1501

Nadler LM, Anderson KC, Marti G, Bates MP, Park E, Daley JF, Schlossman SF (1983) B4, a human B lymphocyte-associated antigen expressed on normal, mitogen-activated, and malignant B-lymphocytes. J Immunol 131:244–250

O'Connor R, Liu C, Ferris CA, Guild BC, Teicher BA, Corvi C, Liu Y, Arceci RJ, Goldmacher VS, Lambert JM, Blattler WA (1995) anti-B4-blocked ricin synergizes with doxorubicin and etoposide on multidrug-resistant and drug-sensitive tumors. Blood 86:4286–4294

Pai LH, Bookman MA, Ozols RF, Young RC, Smith JW II, Longo DL, Gould B, Frankel A, McClay EF, Howell S, Reed E, Willingham MC, Fitzgerald DJ, Pastan I (1991) Clinical evaluation of intraperitoneal Pseudomonas exotoxin immunoconjugate of OVB3-PE in patients with ovarian cancer. J Clin Oncol 9:2095–2103

Parker SL, Tong T, Bolden S, Wingo PA (1996) Cancer statistics 1996. CA Cancer J Clin 46:5–27

Philip T, Guglielmi C, Hagenbeek A, Somers R, Van Der Lelie H, Bron D, Sonneveld P, Gisselbrecht C, Cahn J-Y, Harousseau J-L, Coiffier B, Biron P, Mandelli F, Chauvin F (1995) Autologous bone marrow transplantation as compared with salvage chemotherapy in relapses of chemotherapy-sensitive non-Hodgkin's lymphoma. N Engl J Med 333:1540–1545

Pluda JM, Yarchoan R, Jaffe ES, Feuerstein IM, Solomon D, Steinberg SM, Wyvill KM, Raubitschek A, Katz D, Broder S (1990) Development of non-Hodgkin's lymphoma in a cohort of patients with severe human immunodeficiency virus (HIV) infection on long-term anti retroviral therapy. Ann Intern Med 113:276–282

Robertson MJ, Roy DC, Soiffer R, Belanger R, Gyger M, Perreault C, Anderson K, Freedman A, Nadler LM, Ritz J (1993) More rapid engraftment after infusion of autologous bone marrow treated with anti-My9-blocked ricin compared to bone marrow treated with Ant-My9 and complement. Blood 82:640a

Roy DC, Griffin JD, Belvin M, Blattler WA, Lambert JM, Ritz J (1991) anti-My9-blocked ricin: an immunotoxin for selective targeting of acute myeloid leukemia cells. Blood 77:2404–2412

Roy DC, Robertson MJ, Belanger R, Gyger M, Perreault C, Bonny Y, Soiffer R, Epstein C, Esseltine D, Ritz J (1993) Update on anti-My9-bR depleted autologous bone marrow transplantation for patients with acute myeloid leukemia. XVIIIth congress of the Association of Hematologists-Oncologists of Quebec

Roy DC, Belanger R, Perrault C, Bonny Y, Busque L, Kassis J, Boileau J, Lavalee R, Guertin MJ, D'Angelo G, Esseltine D, Gyger M (1995a) High dose therapy in non-Hodgkin's lymphoma using anti-B4-bR immunotoxin purging. 4th international symposium on immunotoxins, Myrtle Beach, SC

Roy DC, Perreault C, Belanger R, Gyger M, Le Houillier C, Blattler WA, Lambert JM, Ritz J (1995b) Elimination of B-lineage leukemia and lymphoma cells from bone marrow grafts using anti-B4-blocked ricin immunotoxin. J Clin Immunol 15:51–57

Salmon SE, Cassady JR (1993) Plasma cell neoplasms. In: Devita VT Jr, Hellman S, Rosenberg SA (eds) Cancer: principles and practice of oncology, fourth edition. Lippincott, Philadelphia

Scadden DT, Doweiko J, Schenkein D, Bernstein Z, Levine AM, Bresnahan J, Gere J, Esseltine D, Epstein CA (1993) A phase I/II trial of combined immunoconjugate and chemotherapy for AIDS-related lymphoma. Blood 82[Suppl 1]:386a

Szatrowski TP, Larson RA, George S, Dodge R, Hurd D, Kolitz J, Velez-Garcia E, Sklar J, Reynolds C, Westbrook CA, Frankel SR, Stewart C, Bloomfield CD, Schiffer CA (1995) anti-B4-blocked Ricin as consolidation therapy for patients with B-lineage acute lymphoblastic leukemia (ALL): a phase II trial (CALGB 9311). Blood 86[Suppl 1]:783a

Tulpule A, Anderson LJJ, Levine AM, Espina B, Esplin J, Boswell W, Scadden D, Esseltine D, Epstein CL (1994) anti-B4 (CD19) monoclonal antibody conjugated with ricin (B4-blocked ricin: B4bR) in refractory AIDS lymphoma. Proc Am Soc Clin Oncol 13:52

Vitetta ES, Fulton RJ, May RD, Till M, Uhr J (1987) Redesigning nature's poisons to create anti-tumor reagents. Science 238:1098–1104

Vitetta ES, Stone M, Amlot P, Fay J, May R, Till M, Newman J, Clark P, Collins R, Cunningham D, Ghetie V, Uhr JW, Thorpe PE (1991) Phase I immunotoxin trial in patients with B cell lymphoma. Cancer Res 51:4052–4058

Weiss LM, Warnke RA, Sklar J, Cleary ML (1987) Molecular analysis of the t(14;18) chromosomal translocation in malignant lymphomas. N Engl J Med 317:1185–1189

Yunis JJ, Oken MM, Kaplan ME, Ensrud KM, Howe RR (1982) Distinctive chromosomal abnormalities in histological subtypes of non-Hodgkin's lymphoma. N Engl J Med 307:1231–1236

Saporin Immunotoxins

D.J. Flavell

The majority of clinical trials with immunotoxins (ITs) have been conducted with conjugates containing ricin A-chain (Amlot et al. 1993; Grossbard et al. 1992; Vitetta et al. 1991). This has arisen largely as an historical accident simply because the early development of ITs was carried out with ricin as the toxin of choice, for no better reason than its availability. Native ricin poses a major handling hazard requiring special precautions. This is so because ricin is comprised of two chains, an A-chain which possesses the catalytic ribosome inactivating activity and a B-chain which has a lectin-like activity binding to galactose on the cell surface and it is this which confers nonspecific binding and hence toxicity to the intact toxin. Both the A- and B-chains of ricin are glycosylated, which confers liver binding properties that significantly contribute to their hepatotoxicity when used in patients. Saporin, by contrast, is a single chain, ribosome inactivating protein (rip) which consequently has no lectin-like binding activity and moreover is not glycosylated in the native form (Stirpe et al. 1983). Saporin is therefore very considerably safer to handle and can be used in its native form without the attendant toxicities associated with unmodified ricin based immunoconjugates. The seeds of the soapwort plant (*Saponaria officinalis*) are a rich source of saporin and constitutes almost half a percent of the total weight of the seed. The gene for the SO6 isoform of saporin has been cloned and expressed in bacteria (Barthelemy et al. 1993). Saporin, like ricin A-chain, acts as an N-glycosidase catalytically cleaving 28S ribosomal RNA at A-4324 thus irreversibly inactivating cellular ribosome capability (Endo 1988). Despite the fact that saporin and ricin A-chain possess exactly the same catalytic activity and are comparable in their potency, the two proteins are antigenically unrelated.

ITs that deliver saporin (and other toxins) to a selected cell population do so through the specificity of the antibody component . Changing the antibody changes the specificity of the IT target so that ITs may be customised for individual target tumours, providing an appropriate target antigen and respective antibody is available. Anecdotally and by indirect comparison of in vitro performance reported in the literature, immunotoxins constructed with saporin would appear to be at least as potent as those constructed with ricin A-chain, though no formal studies have been published that have made such a direct comparison. With conventional

---

The Simon Flavell Leukaemia Research Unit, University Department of Pathology, Southampton General Hospital, Southampton, Hampshire SO16 6YD, UK

chemically constructed immunoconjugates the nature of the covalent bond between antibody and toxin has been an issue that has led some working with ricin A-chain immunoconjugates to utilise a so called "hindered" disulphide bond as the linker as opposed to a nonhindered disulphide linker (THORPE et al. 1987b). Here the disulphide bond is sterically hindered by side groups rendering this bond less susceptible to reduction in vivo by glutathione-type enzymes. The advantage claimed here is an increased longevity of survival of IT in the circulation and hence a prolongation of exposure of target tumour cells to the drug (THORPE et al. 1987a, 1988). However with the rips saporin and pokeweed anti-viral protein (PAP) there does not appear to be any advantage in constructing the IT with a hindered disulphide bond, either in terms of pharmacokinetics or therapy outcome in preclinical studies in mouse models of human leukaemia and lymphoma (FLAVELL et al. 1994; UCKUN et al. 1993). Hence clinical trials in humans with saporin or PAP based ITs are being conducted with ITs constructed with conventional unhindered disulphide bonds.

There have been several preclinical studies which point to a promising activity of saporin ITs in a variety of human haematological tumours. Earlier studies have reported selective in vitro (BARBIERI et al. 1989a,b; BREGNI et al. 1989; DINOTA et al. 1990; TAZZARI et al. 1992, 1993) activity and more recent work in vivo activity in animal models (FLAVELL et al. 1994, 1995b; MORLAND et al. 1994; PASQUALUCCI et al. 1995) of human leukaemia and lymphoma. The two notable preclinical studies which have now led to clinical trials include an anti-CD30 saporin IT for Hodgkin's disease and anaplastic large cell lymphoma (PASQUALUCCI et al. 1995), and the anti-CD19 IT BU12-SAPORIN for B-lineage acute lymphoblastic leukaemia and non-Hodgkins lymphoma (FLAVELL et al. 1995b).

There is currently only very limited clinical experience with saporin ITs. Studies that are currently being conducted are exclusively aimed at patients with haematological malignancies, in particular Hodgkin's lymphoma and low grade non-Hodgkin's lymphoma. In the first study with a saporin based IT, FALINI et al. (1992) treated four patients with advanced refractory Hodgkin's lymphoma with the anti-CD30 IT BER-H2/SO6. A dose of IT of 0.8mg/kg was given as either one or two doses as an infusion over 4h. Three patients showed a rapid and substantial reduction in tumour mass (50% to > 75%). There were no major toxicities encountered other than transient elevations in liver enzymes and a transient thrombocytopaenia seen in one patient. The authors of this study claim that vascular leak syndrome was not seen in any of the four patients though one patient did develop oedema with an attendant 5kg weight gain, but without a decrease in serum albumin levels as normally seen with IT-induced VLS. The responses were however transient lasting from between 6 and 10 weeks. All patients developed antibody responses to both the antibody and saporin component parts of the IT. This original series has now been expanded to 12 patients with a reported response rate of 40%.

We are currently conducting a phase I clinical trial with the anti-CD19 IT BU12-saporin at two centres in the UK (Southampton and Leeds) in patients with relapsed/refractory B cell lymphoma. This is a dose escalation study whose primary endpoint is determination of the maximum tolerated dose (MTD). At the time of writing five patients have been treated at dose levels of $30\mu g/m^2$ (3 patients) and $60\mu g/m^2$ per day for 7 days (i.e. total doses of $210\mu g/m^2$ and $420\mu g/m^2$, respectively) given daily as a 1h i.v. infusion. No toxicity has thus far been encountered in any of these patients and interesting minor responses have been noted in one patient treated at $30\mu g/m^2$ (tenderness at disease site involving cervical lymph nodes) and $60\mu g/m^2$ (improved platelet counts). Pharmacokinetic data will eventually be gleaned from this study but is currently not available.

Although not strictly an immunoconjugate, though worthy of mention, is the limited clinical experience reported by FRENCH et al. (1995), who targeted saporin to tumour cells utilising two bispecific antibodies (BsAb) each with anti-CD22 specificity in one arm and anti-saporin specificity in the other in four patients with B cell lymphoma. The BsAb was precomplexed with saporin prior to administration i.v. as a 1h infusion. All four patients showed responses with a reduction of 50% or greater in measurable tumour though the duration of the responses was relatively short, the maximum being 28 days. Toxicities encountered were reported as minor with no apparent sign of vascular leak syndrome.

Most clinical trials with ITs in human leukaemia and lymphoma have demonstrated anti-tumour activity, though in general, with a few notable exceptions, the extent and duration of the responses have been disappointing. This does not necessarily mean that IT therapies for cancer have no role to play, as it must be remembered that of necessity the vast majority of patients so far studied have had bulky end stage disease that has become unresponsive to conventional cytotoxic therapy. Largely for ethical reasons this is the traditional patient group that these types of phase I/II clinical trials are conducted in and as such they are a far from ideal patient population in whom to look for durable responses. The fact that responses have been seen at all in this very poor prognostic group should be viewed as encouraging and demonstrates that real anti-tumour activity does exist and the utility of IT treatment in patients with minimal residual disease would seem an application much more likely to yield beneficial effects.

It has become clear in recent years that the major dose-limiting toxicity seen with any IT is the occurrence of vascular leak syndrome (VLS) above serum IT concentrations of $1\mu g/ml$. Any means that can be found to modulate this toxicity or to alternatively improve the therapeutic index so that IT may be used at a dose level not likely to cause VLS would represent a major step forward for this therapeutic approach. There is recently the suggestion from preclinical data that the use of combination IT therapy might ensure the total ablation of all cells in the tumour (FLAVELL et al. 1995a, 1996; GHETIE et al. 1992). If this eventually translates into an increase in IT therapeutic index, then the use of cocktails of ITs in patients with minimum residual disease following tumour debulking by more conventional methods may very well be a promising way ahead for this type of therapeutic modality. In this context a phase I clinical trial with a two combination anti-CD19-positive anti-CD22-ricin A-chain IT cocktail is currently underway in patients with B cell non-Hodgkin's lymphoma at the National Cancer Institute and a saporin-based three IT cocktail (anti-CD19 /CD22/CD38) phase I clinical trial is currently in the planning (FLAVELL 1996). The next few years should therefore hopefully clearly finally show whether or not there really is a role for IT based therapy in the treatment of human malignancy.

References

Amlot PL, Stone MJ, Cunningham D, Fay J, Newman J, Collins R, May R, McCarthy M, Richardson J, Ghetie V, Ramilo O, Thorpe PE, Whr JW, Vitetta ES (1993) A phase I study of an anti-CD22-deglycosylated ricin A-chain immunotoxin in the treatment of B cell lymphomas resistant to conventional therapy. Blood 82:2624–2633

Barbieri L, Bolognesi A, Dinota A, Lappi DA, Soria M, Tazzari PL, Stirpe F (1989a) Selective killing of $CD4^+$ and $CD8^+$ cells with immunotoxins containing saporin. Scand J Immunol 30:369–372

Barbieri L, Dinota A, Gobbi M, Tazzari PL, Rizzi S, Bontadin A, Lemoli RM, Tura S, Stirpe F (1989b) Immunotoxins containing saporin 6 and monoclonal antibodies recognizing plasma cell-associated antigens: effects on target cells and on normal myeloid precursors (CFU-GM). Eur J Haematol 42:238–245

Barthelemy I, Martineau D, Ong M, Matsunami R, Ling N, Benatti L, Cavallaro U, Soria M, Lappi DA (1993) The expression of saporin, a plant ribosome-inactivating protein from the plant *Saponaria officinalis*, in *Escherichia coli*. J Biol Chem 268:6541–6548

Bregni M, Siena S, Formosa A, Lappi DA, Martineau D, Malavasi F, Dorken B, Bonadonna G, Gianni AM (1989) B cell restricted saporin immunotoxins: activity against B cell lines and chronic lymphocytic leukemia cells. Blood 73:753–762

Dinota A, Tazzari PL, Michieli M, Visani G, Gobbi M, Bontadini A, Tassi C, Fanin R, Damiani D, Grandi M, Pileri S, Bolognesi A, Stirpe F, Baccarani M, Tsuruo T, Tura S (1990) In vitro bone marrow purging of multidrug-resistant cells with a mouse monoclonal antibody directed against M_r 170,000 glycoprotein and a saporin-conjugated anti-mouse antibody. Cancer Res 50:4291–4294

Endo Y (1988) The site of action of six different ribosome inactivating proteins from plants on eukaryotic ribosomes: the RNA N-glycosidase activity of the protein. Biochem Biophys Res Commun 150:1032–1036

Falini B, Bolognesi A, Flenghi L, Tazzari PL, Broe MK, Stein H, Durkop H, Aversa F, Corneli P, Pizzolo G, Barbabietola G, Sabattini E, Pileri S, Matelli MF, Stirpe F (1992) Response of refractory Hodgkin's disease to monoclonal anti-CD30 immunotoxin. Lancet 339:1195–1196

Flavell DJ (1996) 3BIT (Saporin-monoclonal antibody conjugate) 17551. Clin Trials Monitor 5:1

Flavell DJ, Boehm DA, Okayama K, Kohler JA, Flavell SU (1994) Therapy of human T-cell acute lymphoblastic leukaemia in severe combined immunodeficient mice with two different anti-CD7-saporin immunotoxins containing hindered or non-hindered disulphide cross linkers. Int J Cancer 58:407–414

Flavell DJ, Boehm DA, Emery L, Noss A, Ramsay A, Flavell SU (1995a) Therapy of human B cell lymphoma bearing SCID mice is more effective with anti-CD19 and anti-CD38-saporin immunotoxins used in combination than with either immunotoxin used alone. Int J Cancer 62:337–344

Flavell DJ, Flavell SU, Boehm D, Emery L, Noss A, Ling NR, Richardson PR, Hardie D, Wright DH (1995b) Preclinical studies with the anti-CD19-saporin immunotoxin BU12-SAPORIN for the treatment of human B cell tumours. Br J Cancer 72:1373–1379

Flavell DJ, Boehm D, Turner JK, Noss A, Flavell SU (1997) Systemic therapy with 3BIT, a triple combination cocktail of anti-CD19, -CD22 and -CD38-saporin immunotoxins is curative of human B cell lymphoma in SCID mice. Cancer Res (in press)

French RR, Hamblin TJ, Bell AJ, Tutt AL, Glennie MJ (1995) Treatment of B cell lymphomas with combination of bispecific antibodies and saporin. Lancet 346:223–224

Ghetie M-A, Tucker K, Richardson J, Uhr JW, Vitetta ES (1992) The antitumour activity of an anti-CD22 immunotoxin in SCID mice with disseminated daudi lymphoma is enhanced by either an anti-CD19 antibody or an anti-CD19 immunotoxin. Blood 80:2351–2320

Grossbard ML, Freedman AS, Ritz J, Coral F, Goldmacher VS, Eliseo L, Spector N, Dear K, Lambert JM, Blattler WA, Taylor JA, Nadler LM (1992) Serotherapy of B cell neoplasms with anti-B4-blocked ricin. A phase I trial of daily bolus infusion. Blood 79:576–585

Morland BJ, Barley J, Boehm D, Flavell SU, Ghaleb N, Kohler JA, Okayama K, Wilkins B, Flavell DJ (1994) Effectiveness of HB2(anti-CD7)-saporin immunotoxin in an in vivo model of human T-cell leukaemia developed in severe combined immunodeficient mice. Br J Cancer 69:279–285

Pasqualucci L, Wasik M, Teicher BA, Flenghi L, Bolognesi A, Stirpe F, Polito L, Falini B, Kadin ME (1995) Antitumour activity of anti-CD30 immunotoxin (Ber-H2/saporin) in vitro and in severe combined immunodeficiency disease mice xenografted with human CD30$^+$ anaplastic large-cell lymphoma. Blood 85:2139–2146

Stirpe F, Gasperi-Campani G, Barbieri G, Falasca A, Abbondanza A, Stevens WA (1983) Ribosome inactivating proteins from the seeds of saponaria officinalis L (soapwort), of *Agrostemma githago* L (corn cockle) and of *Asparagus officinalis* (asparagus) and from the latex of *Hura crepitans* L (sandbox tree). Biochem J 216:617

Tazzari PL, Bolognesi A, Totero DD, Falini B, Lemoli RM, Soria MR, Pileri S, Gobbi M, Stein H, Flenghi L, Martelli MF, Stirpe F (1992) Ber-H2 (anti-CD30)-saporin immunotoxin: a new tool for the treatment of Hodgkin's disease and CD30+ lymphoma: in vitro evaluation. Br J Haematol 11: 203–211

Tazzari PL, Zhang S, Chen Q, Sforzini S, Bolognesi A, Stirpe F, Xie H, Moretta A, Ferrini S (1993) Targeting of saporin to CD25-positive normal and neoplastic lymphocytes by an anti-saporin/anti-CD25 bispecific monoclonal antibody: in vitro evaluation. Br J Cancer 67:1248–1253

Thorpe PE, Blakey DC, Brown AN, Knowles PP, Knyba RE, Wallace PM, Watson GJ, Wawrzynczak EJ (1987a) Comparison of two anti-thy ll-abrin A-chain immunotoxins prepared with different cross-linking agents: antitumor effects, in vivo fate, and tumor cell mutants. J Natl Cancer Inst 79:1101–1112

Thorpe PE, Wallace PM, Knowles PP et al (1988) Improved anti-tumor effects of immunotoxins prepared with deglycosylated ricin A-chain and hindered disulphide linkages. Cancer Res 48:6396–6403

Thorpe PE, Wallace PM, Knowles PP, Relf MG, Brown ANF, Watson GJ, Knyba RE, Wawrzynczak EJ, Blakey DC (1987b) New coupling agents for the synthesis of immunotoxins containing a hindered disulfide bond with improved stability in vivo. Cancer Res 47:5924–5931

Uckun FM, Myers DE, Irvin JD, Kuebelbeck VM, Finnegan D, Chelstrom LM, Houston LL (1993) Effects of the intermolecular toxin-monoclonal antibody linkage on the in vivo stability, immunogenicity and anti-leukemic activity of B43 (anti-CDl9) pokeweed antiviral protein immunotoxin. Leuk Lymph 9:459–476

Vitetta ES, Stone M, Amlot P, Fay J, May R, Till M, Newman J, Clark P, Collins R, Cunningham D, Ghetie V, Uhr JW, Thorpe PE (1991) Phase I immunotoxin trial in patients with B cell lymphoma. Cancer Res 51:4052–4058

Diphtheria Toxin Fusion Proteins

F.M. Foss[1], M.N. Saleh[2], J.G. Krueger[3], J.C. Nichols,[4] and J.R. Murphy[1]

1	Introduction	63
2	Diphtheria Toxin	64
3	Construction of the Diphtheria Toxin Fusion Proteins	66
4	The Interleukin-2 Fusion Proteins	67
4.1	The $DAB_{486}IL$-2 Fusion Protein	67
4.2	$DAB_{486}IL$-2 Clinical Studies	67
4.3	Construction of the $DAB_{389}IL$-2 Fusion Protein	69
4.4	Clinical Studies of $DAB_{389}IL$-2 in Lymphoma	69
4.5	Application of $DAB_{389}IL$-2 to Lymphocyte-Mediated Cutaneous Diseases	76
References		77

1 Introduction

Two different approaches have been undertaken to develop targeted biomolecules for therapeutics. The first was the construction of immunotoxins consisting of monoclonal antibodies chemically linked through a disulfide bond to a plant or bacterial toxin or radionuclide. Instability of the chemical conjugation of some of the earlier immunotoxins led to the concept of using protein engineering and recombinant DNA to assemble fusion genes combining the sequences for the enzymatically active and translocation domains of a toxin with those of a specific targeting ligand. From the outset, the prospect of using recombinant DNA methods to assemble the structural genes encoding bacterial toxin growth factor fusion toxins, or fusion proteins, offered significant advantages over chemical conjugation in the assembly of chimeric proteins. Most importantly, the fusion junction, or point at which the substitute receptor binding domain was linked to the toxin fragment, could be precisely determined. Expression of the fusion gene in recombinant *Escherichia coli* would then result in the synthesis of a single homo-

---

[1] Boston University Medical Center, 88 East Newton Street, Evans Bldg, Room 556 Boston, MA 02118, USA
[2] Department of Medicine, University of Alabama School of Medicine, Birmingham, AL, USA
[3] Laboratory of Investigative Dermatology, Rockefeller University, New York, NY, USA
[4] Seragen, Inc., Hopkinton, MA, USA

geneous gene product rather than the mixture of isomeric forms which result from the chemical conjugation process used in the generation of immunotoxins, thereby leading to a theoretically more uniform agent for clinical studies.

A number of years ago, Murphy and colleagues explored the use of diphtheria toxin as a platform for the development of genetically engineered toxins, in which substitution of the native receptor binding domain with specific growth factors would result in a family of biologically active fusion proteins. These "new" toxins would combine the potent cytotoxic active of diphtheria toxin with the cell receptor specificity of the growth factor employed as the substitute receptor binding domain, creating a targeted therapeutic agent for human disease.

2 Diphtheria Toxin

The choice of diphtheria toxin as the toxophore for receptor binding domain substitution was based upon a detailed understanding of the structure-function relationship of the molecule. In their classic study, Uchida, Gill, and Pappenheimer (UCHIDA et al. 1971) demonstrated that the structural gene for diphtheria toxin was carried by corynebacteriophage β. This study also provided the foundation for subsequent studies on the structure function relationships of diphtheria toxin by demonstrating that the enzymatically active A fragment was positioned on the NH_2-terminal end of the toxin, whereas the receptor binding domain of the toxin was carried on fragment B. Shortly thereafter, MURPHY et al. (1974) used β-phage DNA to program S-30 extracts of *E. coli* and demonstrated, in this coupled transcription translation system, that biologically active diphtheria toxin could be synthesized in vitro.

It was known quite early that native diphtheria toxin was a three domain protein consisting of the enzymatically active domain (fragment A), the hydrophobic domain (NH_2-terminal portion of fragment B), and the receptor binding domain (COOH-terminal portion of fragment B). The process by which diphtheria toxin intoxicates sensitive eukaryotic cells involves at least the following steps, as shown in Fig. 1: (1) binding of the toxin to its cell surface receptor, (2) activation of the catalytic domain by a proteolytic cleavage ("nicking") of the toxin in a sensitive exposed 14 amino acid loop that is subtended by Cys-186 and Cys-201, (3) internalization of the bound toxin into endosomes by receptor-mediated endocytosis, and following acidification of the endocytic vesicle, (4) the facilitated delivery of the catalytic domain across the endocytic vesicle membrane and into the cytosol. Once delivered to the cytosol, fragment A rapidly catalyzes the adenosine diphosphate ribosylation of elongation factor 2 which results in the inhibition of protein synthesis and subsequent death of the cell.

The first step in the intoxication process is the specific binding of diphtheria toxin to its cell surface receptor. MIDDLEBROOK et al. (1978) were able to correlate the apparent sensitivity of a given cell line to diphtheria toxin with the number of

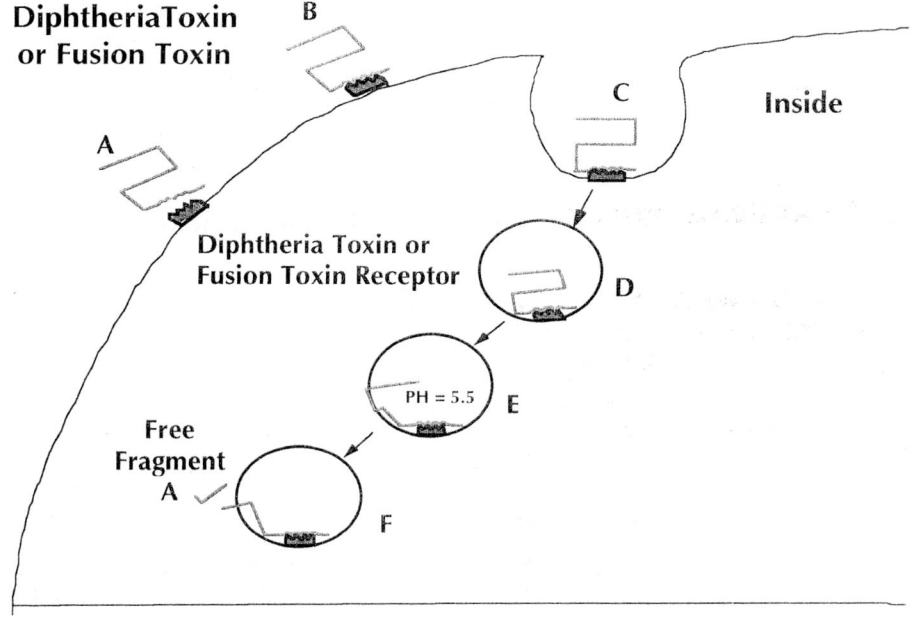

Fig. 1. Mechanism of action of diphtheria toxin. Diphtheria toxin recognizes its receptor on the cell surface (*A*). The receptor-binding domain of the toxin binds to the cell surface receptor (*B*). The toxin-receptor complex is internalized (*C*) by receptor-mediated endocytosis into endosomal vesicles (*D*). The vesicles undergo acidification, resulting in a conformational change in the transmembrane domain of the toxin which allows it to insert into the vesicle membrane and induce pore formation (*E*). Delivery of free fragment A, the enzymatically active part of the toxin, into the cytoplasm (*F*)

receptors on the cell surface. The initial localization of the diphtheria toxin receptor binding domain to the COOH-terminal region of fragment B was based upon the findings that CRM45, a premature chain termination mutant of the toxin which lacked the COOH-terminal 15,000 dalton region, failed to bind to the diphtheria toxin receptor and block the toxic activity of diphtheria toxin on cells (UCHIDA et al. 1971, 1973). In addition, observations made by many investigators using different approaches strongly suggested that the functional native receptor binding domain was positioned in the COOH-terminal 50 amino acids of the toxin (HAYAKAWA et al. 1983; MURPHY et al. 1986; GREENFIELD et al. 1987; MYERS and VILLEMEZ 1988; ROLF and EIDELS 1993).

Once diphtheria toxin is bound to its cell surface receptor, it is internalized into the cell by receptor-mediated endocytosis (MOYA et al. 1985; MORRIS et al. 1985). Early endocytic vesicles are known to be acidified by specific vesicular ATPases to an average pH value of 6.2 (FUCHS et al. 1989; CAIN et al. 1989). It is well known that diphtheria toxin must pass through an acidic compartment in order to deliver the catalytic domain to the cytosol. Over a decade ago, it was recognized that under acidic conditions diphtheria toxin and CRM45 will spontaneously insert into the plane of lipid bilayers and form channels (KAGAN et al. 1981; DONOVAN et al. 1981). Moreover, the diameter of the channel has been reported to be 18 Å (KAGAN et al.

1981; HOCH et al. 1985), which is large enough for a denatured, extended fragment A to pass through and be delivered to the cytosol. Importantly, diphtheria toxin-induced channels have been observed in both Vero and CHO cell membranes following a low pH pulse (PAPINI et al. 1988; SANDVIG and OLSNES 1988).

3 Construction of the Diphtheria Toxin Fusion Proteins

MURPHY et al. (1986) described the construction and properties of the first diphtheria toxin fusion protein, $DAB_{486}\alpha$-MSH, in which the native diphtheria toxin receptor binding domain was replaced with α-melanocyte stimulating hormone (α-MSH). This construct employed a unique *Sph*I restriction endonuclease site in the diphtheria toxin structural gene such that amino acid 486 served as the fusion junction between diphtheria toxin-related sequences and α-MSH . Unfortunately, DAB_{486} α-MSH was subject to marked proteolytic degradation in *E. coli*; however, sufficient amounts of the fusion protein were purified to demonstrate specific toxicity for α-MSH receptor bearing cells.

Since the protease(s) sensitive sites of $DAB_{486}\alpha$-MSH appeared to be close to the fusion junction between diphtheria toxin and α-MSH, it was speculated that a fusion protein constructed with a growth factor of larger mass might provide stearic hinderance and thereby minimize degradation. The next fusion proteins synthesized, DAB_{486} IL-2 and DAB_{389} IL-2, utilized interleukin (IL)-2 as a ligand and, as predicted, these larger molecules were largely resistant to proteolysis (WILLIAMS et al. 1987, 1990; BACHA et al. 1988; WATERS et al. 1990). Building on the success with the IL-2 fusion protein constructs, a variety of other growth factors have been used to replace the native receptor binding domain of the toxin, as shown in Table 1. In all instances, these fusion proteins have been shown to be selectively toxic for *only* those eukaryotic cells which express the appropriate cell surface receptor (GREENFIELD et al. 1987; WILLIAMS et al. 1987, 1990; AULLO et al. 1992; LAKKIS et al. 1991; WEN et al. 1991; SHAW et al. 1991; JEAN and MURPHY 1992).

Table 1. Diphtheria toxin-based cell receptor-targeted fusion proteins

Fusion toxin	Receptor	Cytotoxicity (IC_{50})
$DAB_{486}\alpha$-MSH	α-MSH	n.d.
$DAB_{389}\alpha$-MSH	α-MSH	3×10^{-11}M
DAB_{486} IL-2	IL-2	1×10^{-11}M
DAB_{389} IL-2	IL-2	1×10^{-12}M
DAB_{389} mIL-4	IL-4	2×10^{-10}M
DAB_{389} IL-6	IL-6	2×10^{-11}M
DAB_{389} IL-7	IL-7	1×10^{-10}M
DAB_{389} EGF	EGF	1×10^{-11}M
DAB_{389} CD4	HIV gp120	1×10^{-9}M

DAB, diphtheria toxin fusion protein; MSH, melanocyte-stimulating hormone; IL, interleukin; EGF, epidermal growth factor.

4 The Interleukin-2 Fusion Proteins

4.1 The DAB_{486}IL-2 Fusion Protein

WILLIAMS et al. (1987) described the genetic construction, expression, and purification of the DAB_{486} IL-2 fusion protein. In contrast to α-MSH, the DAB_{486} IL-2 fusion protein could be readily purified from recombinant *E.coli* in good yield. The purified DAB_{486} IL-2 was biologically active and selectively inhibited protein synthesis in IL-2 receptor bearing cells with an IC_{50} of 10^{-11}M. Cells lacking the IL-2 receptor were resistant to the fusion protein, with IC_{50} of $> 10^{-8}$M. BACHA et al. (1988) demonstrated that receptor binding was required for fusion protein-mediated cytotoxicity.

It has further been shown that cells bearing the high-affinity isoform of the IL-2 receptor (p55, p75, p64) are the most sensitive to intoxication by the IL-2 fusion proteins (WATERS et al. 1990). The early events following binding of DAB_{486} IL-2 to the high affinity receptor have been shown to mimic those of IL-2, with increase in messenger RNAs for IL-2, IL-2 receptor, c-*myc*, and interferon-γ. This initial stimulation is rapidly followed by inhibition of protein synthesis such that by 12h the messenger RNA profiles that of a cell treated with cycloheximide (WALZ et al. 1989). Since the high-affinity form of the receptor (TAKESHITA et al. 1992) is found only on activated proliferating T cells, recently activated B cells, and activated monocytes, and selected leukemia and lymphoma cells (WALDMANN 1986, 1990), the NK cells which constitutively express the intermediate form of the receptor (p75 p64) and selected neoplastic cells expressing only the p55 and p64 components (WEIDMANN et al. 1992) are less sensitive to the action of the fusion protein.

4.2 DAB_{486}IL-2 Clinical Studies

IL-2 receptor expression has been reported on subsets of hematopoietic malignancies, including Hodgkin's disease, low and intermediate grade non-Hodgkin's lymphoma, cutaneous T cell lymphoma, HTLV-1-associated adult T cell leukemia/ lymphoma, and chronic lymphocytic leukemia (CRAIG and BANKS 1992; UCHIYAMA et al. 1985; STRAUCHEN and BREAKSTONE 1987; SHEIBANI et al. 1987; BARNETT et al. 1988; ROSOLEN et al. 1989; KUNG et al. 1988).

A series of phase I/II clinical studies were developed to determine the safety, tolerability, and pharmacokinetics of the first generation IL-2 fusion protein, DAB_{486}IL-2, in patients with refractory hematologic malignancies (LEMAISTRE et al. 1992, 1993; SCHWARTZ et al. 1992; HESKETH et al. 1993; FOSS et al. 1994). In these studies, IL-2 receptor expression was determined based on immunostaining with anti-Tac (CD25) antibody on available tumor tissue of enrolled patients, but detectable IL-2R expression was not required for eligibility due to inaccessibility of fresh tissue in many patients. The initial clinical trials were designed as a three patient cohort dose escalation in which single and multiple doses of the fusion protein were administered by intravenous injection, either as a bolus, or 90 min infusion. The initial dose was 700ng/kg per day and was escalated to 400µg/kg per day. Adverse effects were generally mild and included nausea/vomiting, hypersensitivity, fever/malaise/chills, and elevations in serum hepatic transaminases. The maximal tolerated dose for $DAB_{486}IL$-2 was 400µg/kg per day, above which renal insufficiency occurred. All of the adverse effects observed in these studies were transient, not cumulative, and did not preclude repeated administration of the fusion protein to patients who responded to therapy. In addition, there were no changes in circulating normal lymphocyte subsets during or following therapy, and no increased incidence of opportunistic infection was observed.

The time course of analysis of $DAB_{486}IL$-2 concentrations in serum, using a nonlinear mathematical model, showed that the clearance of the fusion protein followed a one-component model with a $t_{1/2}$ of approximately 11 min at dose levels of 200–400µg/kg (LeMaistre et al. 1993). Moreover, the pharmacokinetics of the fusion protein did not change following multiple courses of administration.

In many patients increased serum levels of soluble IL-2 receptor (sIL-2R) were detected; however, there was no correlation between the clearance rates of the fusion protein from circulation and the level of sIL-2R. Bacha (personal communication) had found previously that the presence of 50,000 units/ml of sIL-2R failed to inhibit the cytotoxic action of $DAB_{486}IL$-2 in vitro. Following administration of $DAB_{486}IL$-2, approximately 60% of the patients had an anamnestic response to the diphtheria toxin component of the fusion protein. Few patients, however, had anti-IL-2 titers prior to study entry. After one or more course of fusion protein administration approximately half of the patients developed low titers of anti-IL-2 antibodies. As was seen with sIL-2R, the presence of either antidiphtheria toxin-related or anti-IL-2 antibodies did not appear to prevent an antitumor response.

Clinical responses were seen in these phase I studies in patients with low and intermediate grade non-Hodgkin's lymphoma, Hodgkin's disease, and cutaneous T cell lymphoma, as shown in Table 2. All of these patients had refractory disease and had failed at least two prior chemotherapy regimens. While IL-2 receptor expression on the patient's tumor tissue was not a requirement for entry onto this study, immunohistochemical studies were performed in patients in whom tissue was readily accessible for biopsy. All of the responders had demonstrable IL-2 receptor expression as measured by immunoreactivity with the CD25 (anti-Tac) antibody.

Table 2. Clinical response to $DAB_{486}IL$-2

Diagnosis	Number enrolled	CR	PR	Total CR + PR (%)
NHL	51	1	3	4 (8%)
HD	14	1	0	1 (7%)
CTCL	36	1	5	6 (17%)

DAB, diphtheria toxin fusion protein; IL, interleukin; NHL, non-Hodgkin's lymphoma; HD, Hodgkin's disease; CTCL, cutaneous T cell lymphoma; CR, complete response; PR, partial response.

The most impressive responses in these studies occurred in patients with cutaneous T cell lymphoma. One patient with tumor stage cutaneous T cell lymphoma had a complete remission with disappearance of all of his tumors, and he has remained disease-free without further therapy for at least 5 years (HESKETH et al. 1993). Another patient with diffuse plaque stage disease had significant clearing of his lesions, and two patients with the Sezary syndrome experienced marked improvement in skin exfoliation and pruritus without a significant change in the numbers of circulating Sezary cells (Foss et al. 1994).

4.3 Construction of the DAB$_{389}$IL-2 Fusion Protein

While DAB$_{486}$ IL-2 demonstrated high specific activity in vitro, its half-life was less than 5 min, perhaps due to the propensity of the molecule through hydrophobic interactions to form aggregates in solution. Efforts to reengineer the molecule were undertaken by WILLIAMS and colleagues, who performed a series of experiments in which a series of truncated DAB molecules were created and tested for binding and bioactivity. They demonstrated that the deletion of 97 amino acids from the diphtheria toxin fragment B resulted in a molecule (DAB$_{389}$ IL-2) which had a two- to threefold higher kDa than DAB$_{486}$ IL-2, with resulting tenfold increase in potency (WILLIAMS et al. 1990; KIYOKAWA et al. 1991). Based on these results, it was determined that amino acid 389 of diptheria toxin is the optimal site for the genetic fusion of cell receptor binding ligands. As seen in Fig. 2, the X-ray crystallographic structure of native diphtheria toxin has shown that amino acid 388 (amino acid 389 of the fusion proteins) is positioned at the end of a random coil separating the transmembrane domain from the native receptor binding domain (CHOE et al. 1992). DAB$_{389}$IL-2, like its progenitor, binds to and is selectively cytotoxic only for high-affinity IL-2 receptor bearing cells.

4.4 Clinical Studies of DAB$_{389}$IL-2 in Lymphoma

Because of the encouraging results with DAB$_{486}$IL-2, further clinical studies were performed with the redesigned fusion protein, DAB$_{389}$IL-2. A phase I/II study of DAB$_{389}$IL-2 was initiated in patients with non-Hodgkin's lymphoma, Hodgkin's disease, and cutaneous T cell lymphoma whose tumors expressed the IL-2 receptor as determined by immunohistochemical staining using the anti-CD25 antibody and antibodies directed against the p75 component of the IL-2 receptor (LEMAISTRE et al., in press; SALEH et al., in press). Only cells histologically and immunohistochemically representative of malignant cells were assessed for IL-2R. Tumor sections were considered positive if >25% of the tumor cells stained with either p55 or p75. Patients with HIV-associated T cell malignancy were excluded from this study.

A minimum of three patients were studied at each dose level with each patient receiving the same dose for the duration of treatment. A treatment cycle consisted of DAB$_{389}$IL-2 administered over 5 min daily for 5 days. Treatment cycles were

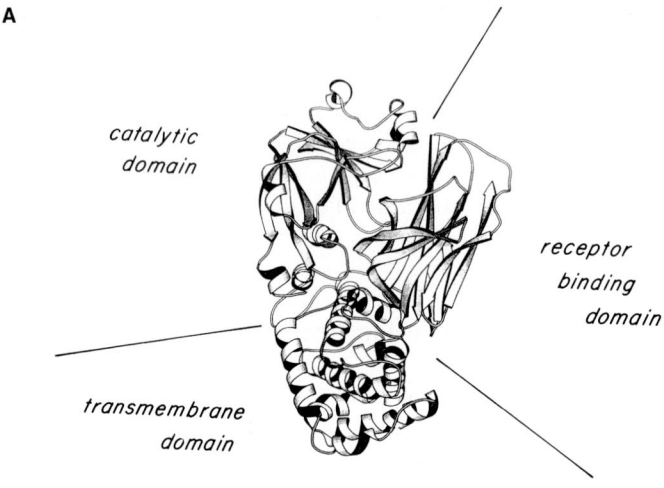

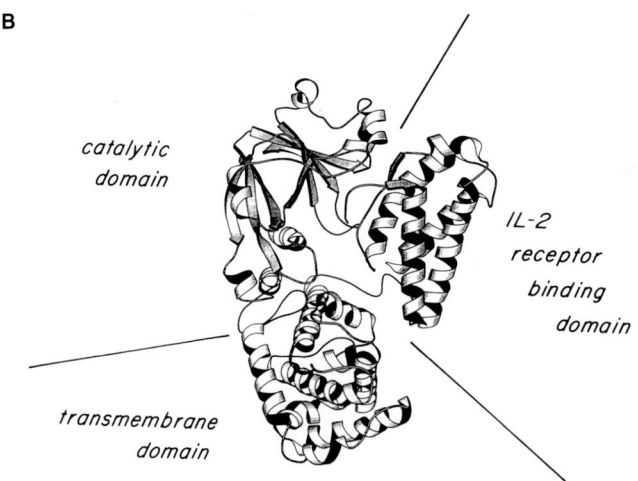

Fig. 2A,B. Ribbon diagram of the X-ray crystal structure of native diphtheria toxin (**A**) (CHOE et al. 1992; BENNETT et al. 1994). The catalytic domain, transmembrane domain, and receptor binding domain are shown. The DAB389 IL-2 fusion toxin was constructed by substitution of the receptor-binding domain with the gene for interleukin-2 (**B**). The ribbon diagrams were generated using MOLESCRIPT (KRAULIS 1991)

repeated every 3 weeks. Tumor assessment was performed every two cycles and patients with objective response or stable disease were permitted to receive additional treatment for up to six cycles. Retreatment was permitted as long as drug related toxicity and/or associated laboratory abnormalities had returned to pretreatment baseline or less than grade 1. During the course of this study, $DAB_{389}IL-2$ dosage was determined in micrograms instead of bioactivity units which were used in studies with DAB_{486} IL-2.

A total of 230 patients were screened for inclusion in to the study. IL-2R was detected on tumor specimen from 109 patients (47%). The prevalence of IL-2R was 41% in patients with non-Hodgkin's lymphoma, 62% in patients with cutaneous T cell lymphoma and 83% in patients with Hodgkin's disease. Seventy-three patients fulfilled the eligibility criteria and were enrolled in this study. This was a heavily pretreated patient population having received a mean of five previous therapies. Twenty-five patients (34%) with lymphoma had undergone bone marrow transplantation. Patients received doses ranging from 3 to 31µg/kg per day daily for 5 days. Fifty-two patients (71%) completed two courses and 39 (53%) received three of the six treatments. Overall, one quarter of the patients completed all six cycles of therapy. Thirty-nine patients (53%) discontinued treatment because of disease progression while 12 (16%) patients came off study because of toxicity.

The most common side effect associated with $DAB_{389}IL-2$ was treatment-associated fever/chills (74%), which were self limited or readily reversible with symptomatic treatment. Approximately half of the patients also experienced nausea/vomiting, asthenia and hypotension. The severity of adverse events diminished with subsequent courses and 84 of 91 (92%) of grade 3–4 toxicities occurred during the first or second treatment cycle. Treatment-associated laboratory abnormalities consisted of decreased serum albumin (80%) and reversible elevation of serum transaminases (62%). The association of hypoalbuminemia, hypotension and edema was observed in eight patients with cutaneous T cell lymphoma and was felt to potentially represent a form of mild vascular leak syndrome previously reported with ricin and *Pseudomonas* exotoxin-based immunotoxins. Dose limiting toxicity was observed at the 31µg/kg per day dose and consisted of severe fatigue and asthenia precluding administration of more than one cycle in four of five patients at the dose level. No particular laboratory finding could be linked to this clinical event except for a twofold increase in transaminase elevation compared to the previous dose level (23–27µg/kg per day). Toxicity was reversible in all patients. As shown in Fig. 3, there was no change in circulating populations of T cell subsets or B cells during the course of therapy.

The kinetics of $DAB_{389}IL-2$ best fit a one compartment model with an overall half-life of 72min. The area under the curve (AUC) increased with administered dose. Approximately 38% of the patients demonstrated preexisting antibodies to $DAB_{389}IL-2$ and antibodies were detected in 92% of the study population following two cycles of treatment. Importantly, however, preexisting antibody or antibody development following treatment did not appear to interfere with clinical response or significantly contributed to the side effect profile.

Objective clinical responses were observed in 16 of the 73 patients (22%), including six complete and ten partial responses. Of 35 cutaneous T cell lymphoma patients, 13 (37%) and three of 17 non-Hodgkin's lymphoma patients (18%) demonstrated an objective clinical response. There were no responders in the Hodgkin's disease patients. The median time to response was 2 months (two cycles

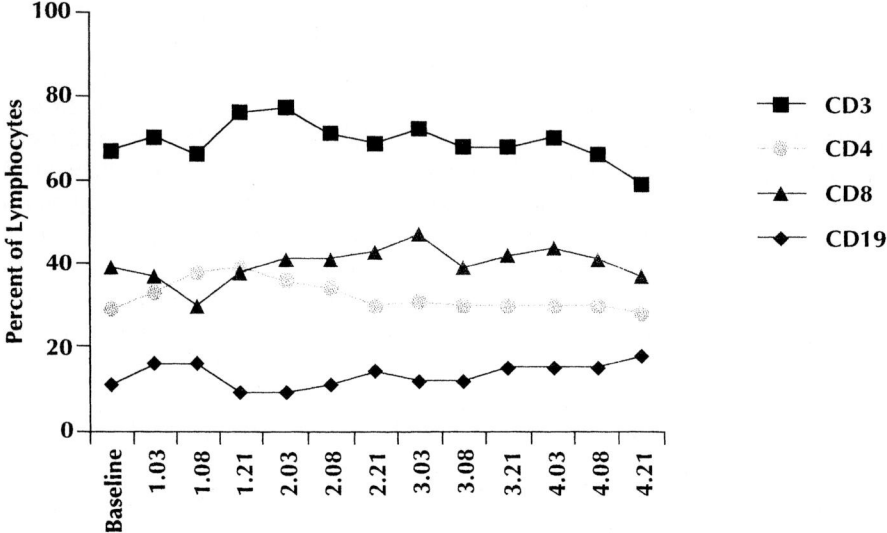

Fig. 3. Lymphocyte subsets during therapy with $DAB_{389}IL$-2. Populations of circulating normal lymphocytes were measured during therapy with $DAB_{389}IL$-2 by flow cytometry on days 3, 8, and 21 of each 21 day cycle for four cycles. Data represents mean for all patients without circulating neoplastic cells (11 non-Hodgkin's disease, 21 Hodgkin's disease). The x-axis shows cycle number and day; the y-axis shows mean % positive cells derived by flow cytometry using antibodies to CD3, CD4, CD8, and CD19 in separate analyses

of treatment) with the median duration of response being 10 months. The most dramatic responses, including five of six complete responses, were observed in patients with cutaneous T cell lymphoma. Four of the five complete responders had failed prior photophoresis. An impressive complete response was achieved in a patient with extensive erythroderm (T4) and palpable adenopathy (stage III). The patient had debilitating plaque disease involving both hands and arms resulting in palmar contractures bilaterally (Fig. 4A,B). He had previously failed photophoresis and PUVA therapy. He was treated at the 15µg/kg per day dose and objective response was documented following four cycles and biopsy proven complete response following six cycles of $DAB_{389}IL$-2. The complete response lasted 16 months. A second patient with extensive tumors measuring 2–3cm involving the entire body including palmar and plantar surface (stage IIb) demonstrated a remarkable clinical response (Fig. 4C–F). He had previously failed topical therapy, phototherapy, chemotherapy, interferon and local radiotherapy. He experienced dramatic shrinkage of tumors following one cycle of treatment at the 27µg/kg per day dose and complete regression of all visible lesions by the end of the second cycle. Complete response was confirmed by biopsy following the fourth cycle. The patient had an unmaintained complete response for 12 months. One patient with primary refractory non-Hodgkin's lymphoma, who had failed bone marrow transplantation, achieved a complete response which has been ongoing for greater than 39 months. Clinical responses were seen at all dose levels.

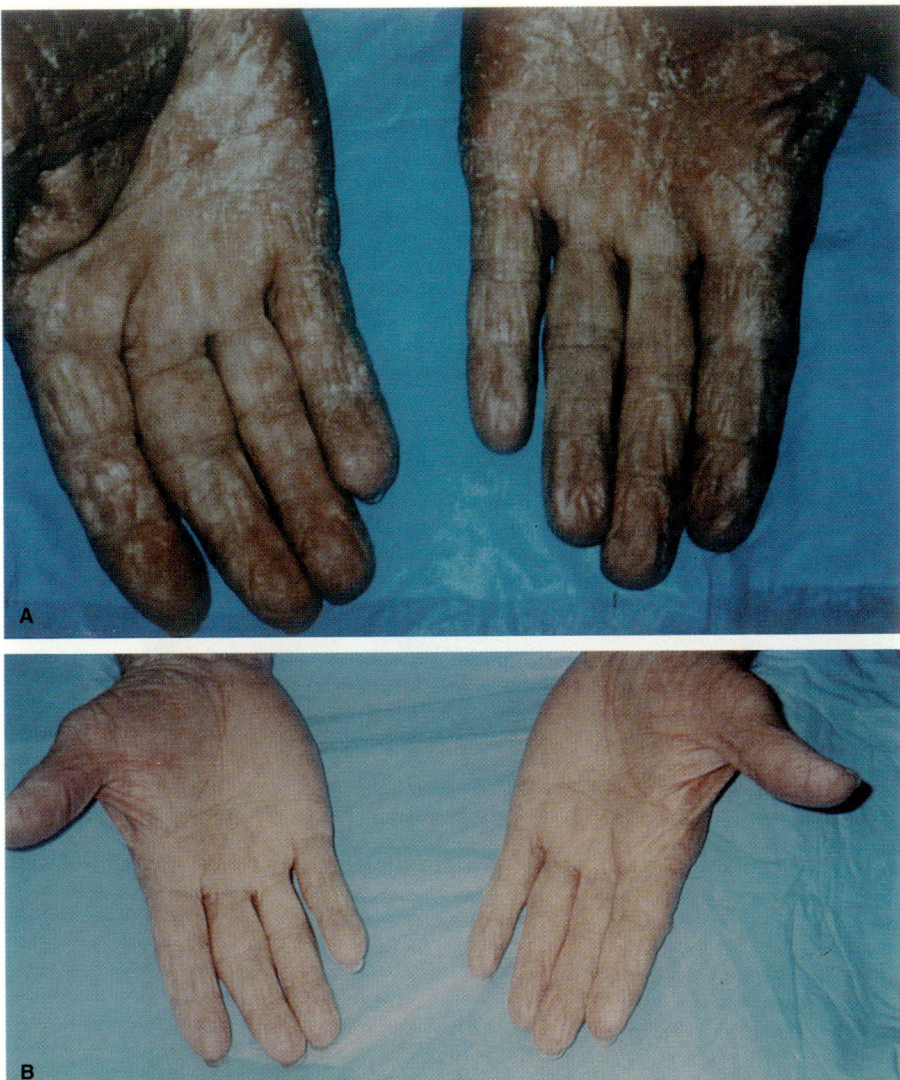

Fig. 4A–F. Clinical response to DAB$_{389}$IL-2. **A, B** Patient with stage III cutaneous T cell lymphoma and Sezary syndrome before (**A**) and after (**B**) four cycles of therapy. The patient achieved a clinical complete response for 16 months. **C–F** Photographs of patient with stage IIb cutaneous T cell lymphoma with diffuse cutaneous tumors before (**C, E**) and after (**D, F**) four cycles of therapy. The patient had a complete response for 12 months

Table 3 compares results from this phase I study with those from the DAB$_{486}$IL-2 studies. The half-life of DAB$_{389}$-IL2 is substantially longer than that of the first generation molecule. Both molecules cause reversible elevation of liver function enzymes though the toxicity profile at maximum tolerated dose (MTD) is

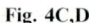

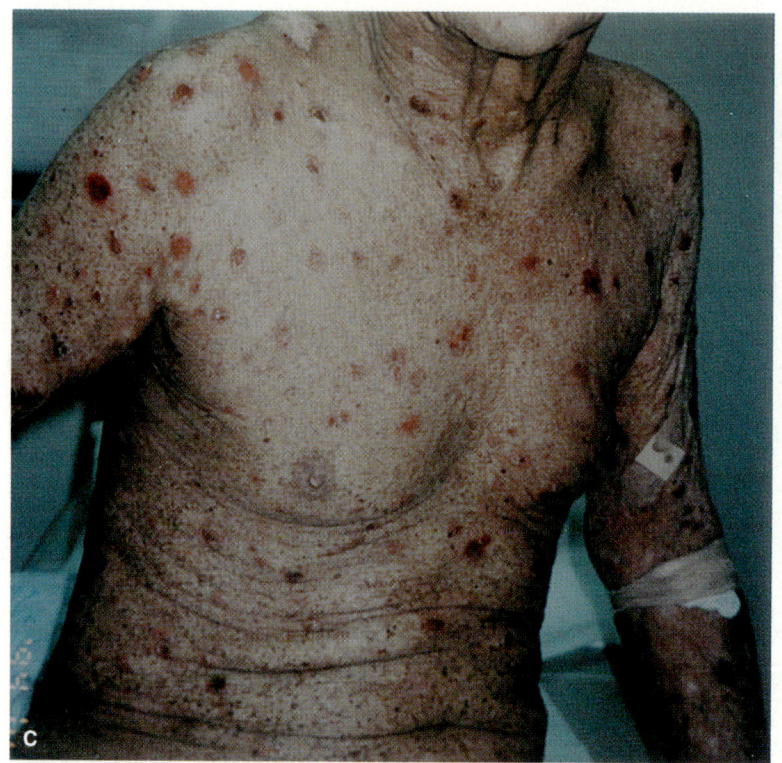

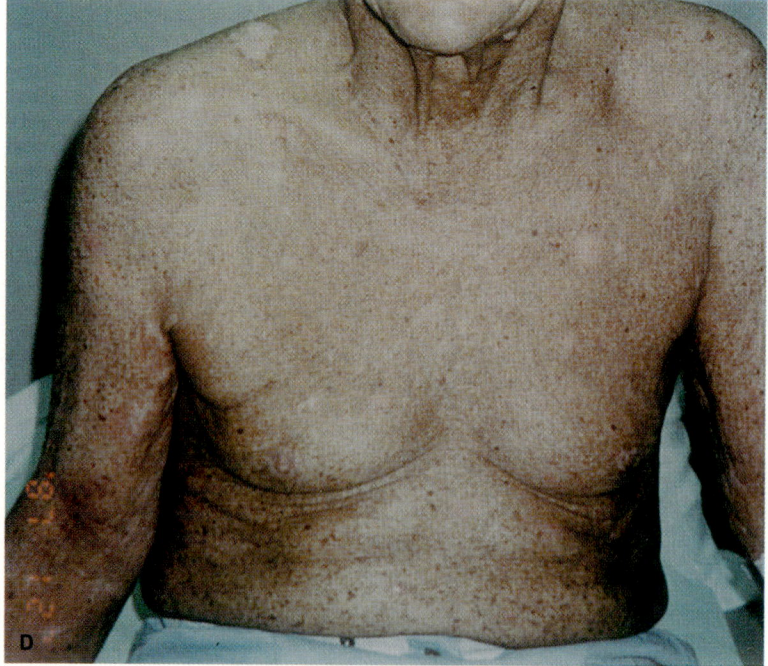

Fig. 4C,D

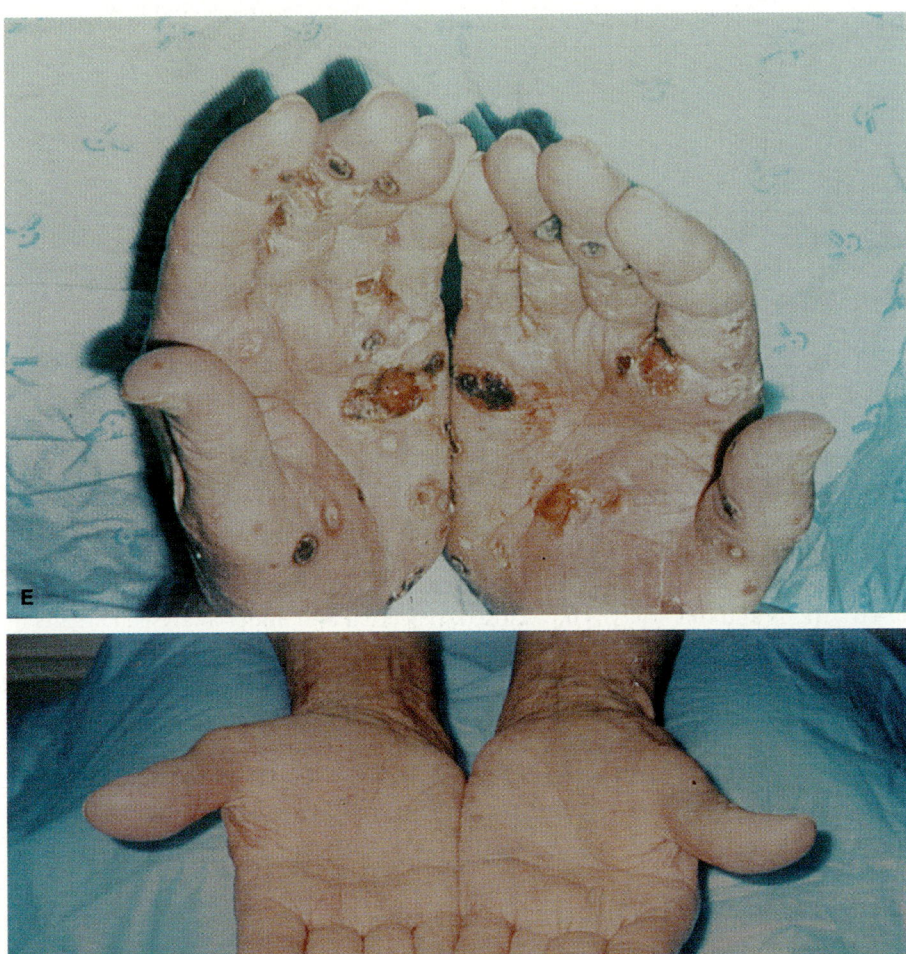

Fig. 4E,F

different for the two reagents. The achievement of objective anti-tumor responses, including durable complete remissions, in a heavily pretreated patient population in this dose escalation study of $DAB_{389}IL-2$ provides compelling evidence for the anti-tumor potential of IL-2 fusion proteins in patients with cutaneous T cell lymphoma. Unlike the experience with most conventional modalities, the complete responses achieved with $DAB_{389}IL-2$ have been durable in the absence of continual or prolonged maintenance therapy. In vitro studies have demonstrated that

Table 3. Comparison of clinical activity of DAB486IL-2 and DAB389-IL-2

	DAB486-IL2	DAB389-IL-2
MTD	300µg/kg per day × 5 days	27µg/kg per day × 5 days
$t_{1/2}$ (min)	11.5 + 4.3	65 + 50
DLT	Renal	Asthenia
Response	11/101(11%)	16/73 (22%)

MTD, maximum tolerated dose; DLT, dose-limiting toxicity.

inhibition of protein synthesis and cell kill can be induced by $DAB_{389}IL$-2 at concentrations as low as 0.1ng/ml and drug exposure time of less than 5min. Kinetic data emerging from this phase I study reveal that comparable biologically active levels of $DAB_{389}IL$-2 are achieved in vivo using the current schedule. It is unclear why responses were not observed in Hodgkin's disease patients in this study, although this may be related to an internalization defect related to lack of expression of all components of the high affinity IL-2 receptor.

Based upon these observations, two phase III clinical trials were initiated using $DAB_{389}IL$-2 in the treatment of cutaneous T cell lymphoma. The first study for refractory patients was an open label treatment study comparing two doses of $DAB_{389}IL$-2, and this study is now closed to accrual and under analysis. Patients in this study were randomized to either 18µg/kg per day or 9µg/kg per day of $DAB_{389}IL$-2 using the phase I/II dosing regimen of five consecutive daily doses every 21 days. The second study, which is still accruing patients, is a double-blind, randomized, placebo-controlled study in earlier stage cutaneous T cell lymphoma patients who have not received prior systemic therapy. In this study, patients will be randomized to placebo or to either the 18µg/kg per day or 9µg/kg per day dose of $DAB_{389}IL$-2.

4.5 Application of $DAB_{389}IL$-2 to Lymphocyte-Mediated Cutaneous Diseases

One important function of the skin is to provide an immunologic barrier to the environment. In normal skin, the epidermal Langerhans cell and the dermal dendritic cell are resident antigen-presenting cells, while T lymphocytes and other immunocytes regularly traffic throughout the epidermis and dermis. Not surprisingly, a wide array of cutaneous diseases are related to local immune activation in skin, to systemic immune activation visible in the skin, or to homing of neoplastic T lymphocytes to the skin. Some immune events, e.g., contact dermatitis to a topical allergen or a drug "rash" due to a systemic medication, are self-limited and are most appropriately treated with short-duration immunosuppressives such as corticosteroids. In contrast a number of autoimmune or inflammatory skin diseases are caused by persistent infiltration of CD4+ or CD8+ T lymphocytes in the epidermis or dermis. Common examples of chronic inflammatory diseases are psoriasis, atopic eczema, lichen planus, alopecia areata, and graft-versus-host disease (GVHD) (following bone marrow transplantation). In each of these conditions, a direct link between activated T lymphocytes and the disease phenotype is suggested by impressive clinical improvements mediated by cyclosporine or other direct immunosuppressives (GUPTA et al. 1990). Each of these conditions represents a considerable therapeutic challenge, as all persist for years, or even a lifetime, and thus require treatment for years-to-decades. Treatment with cyclosporine and other immunosuppressives is usually limited to short periods due to toxicity concerns. Hence, there is significant medical need for alternate treatments, such as to $DAB_{389}IL$-2, which have reduced or non-overlapping toxicity with other available agents.

Presently, only two cutaneous immune-related diseases have been treated with $DAB_{389}IL$-2: cutaneous T cell lymphoma and psoriasis (GOTTLIEB et al. 1995). Psoriasis is considered to be the most common human immune-mediated or autoimmune disease (VYSE and TODD 1996). Its immunological features include: (1) activated antigen-presenting cells in skin lesions, (2) high numbers of T lymphocytes infiltrating affected skin regions, (3) impressive activation of T lymphocytes as measured by expression of the IL-2 receptor α-subunit (CD25), and (4) clonal proliferation of CD8+ T cells in lesional skin (WEINSTEIN and KRUEGER 1993; NICKOLOFF and GRIFFITHS 1990; GOTTLEIB et al. 1986). T cell activation in psoriasis is thought to be driven by an as yet unidentified cutaneous antigen which is presented to T cells by the activated dendritic cells in psoriatic lesions. As pathogenic T lymphocyte clones would control their proliferation through up-regulated "normal" IL-2 receptors, disease-mediating T cell clones should be highly sensitive to $DAB_{389}IL$-2.

While relatively few psoriatic patients have been treated $DAB_{389}IL$-2, this agent has produced remarkable skin clearing or disease improvements in the majority of those treated (GOTTLEIB et al. 1995). Clinical improvement was coupled with reduction in the number of T lymphocytes infiltrating skin lesions and with marked improvement or elimination of keratinocyte hyperproliferation and other cellular aberrations that define the histopathology of psoriasis. While larger series of psoriasis studies are needed, and an optimal dosing regimen for this disease must still be determined, the initial experiments suggest the potential of $DAB_{389}IL$-2 as an effective therapeutic for inflammatory or autoimmune skin disorders. The clinical responsiveness of atopic eczema, alopecia areata, lichen planus, and GVHD to cyclosporine and other immunosuppressives suggests that these diseases are also logical candidates for $DAB_{389}IL$-2 therapy. One potential advantage of $DAB_{389}IL$-2 over cyclosporine (and other noncytotoxic agents) is the potential of $DAB_{389}IL$-2 to eliminate pathogenic T lymphocyte clones and thus produce stable disease remission without the need for repetitive or on-going treatment.

5 The Epidermal Growth Factor Fusion Protein

$DAB_{389}EGF$ is a 48kDa fusion protein in which sequences for the human epidermal growth factor (EGF) are combined with the 389 amino acids of diphtheria toxin (SHAW et al. 1991). $DAB_{389}EGF$ selectively binds to the EGF receptor (EGF-R) and is internalized with inhibition of protein synthesis occurring after entry of the toxin portion of the molecule into the cytosol, as described above for the DAB IL-2 fusion proteins. Mammalian cell lines expressing high levels of EGF-R ($> 10^5$ receptors/cell) are uniformly sensitive to $DAB_{389}EGF$ at concentrations in the range of 1×10^{-11} to 5×10^{-10}M. Cells which have fewer than 10^4 EGF-Rs are intoxicated only at concentrations greater than 10^{-9}M.

The EGF-R is a transmembrane glycoprotein which is expressed on normal and transformed cells of epidermal and mesenchymal origin (CARPENTER and CHEN 1990). The receptor is composed of an extracellular domain, a membrane spanning region, and an inner domain which possesses intrinsic protein tyrosine kinase activity. Overexpression of the EGF-R has been described on colorectal, bladder, pancreatic, head and neck, lung, breast, ovarian, and prostate tumors (VEALE et al. 1989; EISBRUCH et al. 1987; STEELE et al. 1990; SMITH et al. 1989; NEAL and MELLON 1992; LEMOINE et al. 1992; BATTAGLIA et al. 1989; BERCHUCK et al. 1991; MORRIS and DODD 1990). The expression of EGF and EGF-R by many of these tumors suggests the existence of an autocrine growth pathway. Elevated EGF-R expression has been associated with poor prognosis and lack of response to conventional therapies (NICHOLSON et al. 1988).

To date, two phase I studies using $DAB_{389}EGF$ have been conducted in patients with EGF-R expressing malignancies (THEODOULOU et al. 1995). Both studies were cohort dose escalation studies, one with 5 consecutive days of dosing and one with episodic dosing on days 1, 8, 9, 15, 16 every 28 days. Fifty-two patients with metastatic disease were enrolled, and the doses evaluated ranged from 0.3 to 15µg/kg per day. Of the enrolled patients, 12% had prostate cancer, 11% gastrointestinal tumors, 9% head and neck, 6% renal cell, and 5% breast cancer.

Toxicities were similar to those seen with $DAB_{389}IL2$ and included reversible hepatic transaminase elevations in 52% of patients on the first course of treatment, decreasing with subsequent courses. Renal toxicity included elevation of serum creatinine in 25% and abnormal urinanalysis findings in 60%. One patient experienced proximal renal tubular acidosis which resolved with electrolyte supplementation. Hypoalbuminemia was noted in 42% of patients. Other toxicities included fever and chills, nausea, blood pressure alterations, and anorexia. The dose-limiting toxicity was renal tubular acidosis in the consecutive dosing schedule at 9µg/kg per day and back and chest pain in the episodic dosing schedule at 15µg/kg per day.

All patients developed antibodies to $DAB_{389}EGF$ and a proportion of patients developed antibodies to EGF. In most patients, these antibodies were neutralizing in vitro, and there was no correlation between antibody titer and clinical response.

One patient with lung cancer had a partial response at the 6µg/kg per day dose level on the episodic schedule, and three patients had stable disease during the 6 months of dosing during the study. Two of these patients had prostatic carcinoma and were dosed at 1.2 and 4.2µg/kg per day on the consecutive schedule, and one had head and neck cancer and received 0.6µg/kg per day on the episodic schedule. Based on these results, a phase I/II study is currently being conducted in patients with non-small cell lung cancer with a starting dose of 6μg/kg per day every other day for three doses, to be repeated every 21 days.

References

Aullo P, Alcani J, Popoff MR, Klatzman DR, Murphy JR, Boquet P (1992) In vitro effects of a recombinant diphtheria-human CD4 fusion toxin on acute and chronically HIV-1 infected cells. EMBO J 12:921–931
Bacha P, Waters C, Williams J, Murphy JR, Strom TB (1988) Interleukin-2 targeted cytotoxicity: selective action of a diphtheria toxin-related interleukin-2 fusion toxin. J Exp Med 167:612–622
Barnett D, Wilson G, Lawrence A, Buckley G (1988) The interleukin-2 receptor and its expression in the acute leukemias and lymphoproliferative disorders. Dis Markers 6:133–139
Battaglia R, Scambia G, Benedetti P, Baiocchi G, Perrone L, Iaocabellli S, Mancuso S (1989) Epidermal growth factor receptor in gynecological malignancies. Gynecol Obstet Invest 27:42
Bennett MJ, Choe S, Eisenberg D (1994) Domain swapping: entangling alliances between proteins. Proc Natl Acad Sci USA 91:3127–3131
Berchuck A, Rodriguez G, Kamel A, Dodge R, Soper J, Clarke-Pearson D, Bast R (1991) Epidermal growth factor receptor expression in normal ovarian epithelium and ovarian cancer. Am J Obstet Gynecol 164:669
Cain CC, Sipe DM, Murphy RF (1989) Regulation of endocytic pH by the Na^+K^+-ATPase in living cells. Proc Natl Acad Sci USA 86:544–548
Carpenter G, Chen S (1990) Epidermal growth factor. J Biol Chem 265:7709
Choe S, Bennett M, Fujii G, Curmi P, Kantardjieff K, Collier R, Eisenberg D (1992) The crystal structure of diphtheria toxin. Nature 357:216–222
Craig F, Banks P (1992) Detection of the alpha and beta components of the interleukin-2 receptor using immunologic techniques. Mod Pathol 5:118a
Donovan JJ, Simon MI, Draper RK, Montal M (1981) Diphtheria toxin forms transmembrane channels in planar lipid bilayers. Proc Natl Acad Sci USA 78:172–176
Eisbruch A, Blick M, Lee J, Sacks P, Gutterman J (1987) Analysis of the epidermal growth factor receptor in fresh human head and neck tumors. Cancer Res 47:3603
Foss F, Borkowski T, Gilliom M, Stetler-Stevenson M, Jaffe E, Tomkins A, Bastian A, Nylen P, Woodworth T, Udey M, Sausville E (1994) Chimeric fusion protein toxin DAB(486)IL2 in refractory mycosis fungoides and the sezary syndrome: correlation of activity and IL2 receptor expression in a phase II study. Blood 84(6):1765–1774
Fuchs R, Schmid S, Mellman I (1989) A possible role for Na^+, K^+-ATPase in regulating ATP-dependent endosome acidification. Proc Natl Acad Sci USA 86:539–543
Gottlieb AB, Lifshitz B, Fu SM, Staiano-Coico L, Wang CY, Carter DM (1986) Expression of HLA-DR molecules by keratinocytes and presence of Langerhans cells in the dermal infiltrate of active psoriatic plaques. J Exp Med 164:1013–1028
Gottlieb SL, Gilleaudeau P, Johnson R, Estes L, Woodworth TG, Gottlieb AB, Krueger JG (1995) Response of psoriasis to a lymphocyte-selective toxin ($DAB_{389}IL$-2) suggests a primary immune, but not keratinocyte, pathogenic basis. Nature Med 1:442–447
Greenfield L, Johnson VG, Youle RJ (1987) Mutations in diphtheria toxin separate binding from entry and amplify immunotoxin selectivity. Science 238:536–539
Gupta AK, Ellis CN, Nickoloff BJ, Goldfarb MT, Ho VC, Rocher LL, Griffiths CEM, Cooper KD, Voorhees JJ (1990) Oral cyclosporine in the treatment of inflammatory and noninflammatory dermatoses. A clinical and immunopathologic analysis. Arch Dermatol 126:339–350
Hayakawa S, Uchida T, Mekada E, Moynihan MR, Okada Y (1983) Monoclonal antibody against diphtheria toxin: effect on toxin binding and entry into cells. J Biol Chem 258:4311–4317
Hesketh P, Caguioa P, Koh H, Dewey H, Facada A, McCaffrey R, Parker K, Nylen P, Woodworth T (1993) Clinical activity of a cytotoxic fusion protein in the treatment of cutaneous T cell lymphoma. J Clin Oncol 11:1628–1690

Hoch DH, Romero-Mira M, Ehrich BE, Finkelstein A, DasGupta BR, Simpson LL (1985) Channels formed by botulinum, tetanus, and diphtheria toxins in planar lipid bilayers: relevance to translocation of proteins across membranes. Proc Natl Acad Sci USA 82:336–343

Jean L-F, Murphy JR (1992) Diphtheria toxin receptor binding domain substitution with interleukin-6: genetic construction and interleukin-6 receptor specific action of a diphtheria toxin-related interleukin-6 fusion protein. Protein Eng 4:989–994

Kagan BL, Finkelstein A, Colombini M (1981) Diphtheria toxin fragment forms large pores in phospholipid bilayer membranes. Proc Natl Acad Sci USA 78:4950–4954

Kiyokawa T, Williams DP, Snider CE, Strom TB, Murphy JR (1991) Protein engineering of diphtheria toxin-related interleukin-2 fusion toxins to increase biologic potency for high affinity interleukin-2 receptor bearing target cells. Protein Eng 4:463–468

Kraulis PJ (1991) MOLESCRIPT: a program to produce both detailed and schematic plots of protein structures. J Appl Crystallogr 24:946–950

Kung E, Meissner K, Loning T (1988) Cutaneous T cell lymphoma: immunocytochemical study on activation/proliferation and differentiation associated antigens in lymph nodes, skin, and peripheral blood. Virchows Arch [A] Pathol Anat 413:539–549

Lakkis F, Steele A, Pacheco-Silva A, Kelley VE, Strom TB, Murphy JR (1991) Interleukin-2 receptor targeted cytotoxicity: genetic construction and properties of diphtheria toxin-related interleukin-4 fusion toxins. Eur J Immunol 21:2253–2258

LeMaistre CF, Meneghetti C, Rosenblum M, Reuben J, Parker K, Shaw J, Woodworth T, Parkinson D (1992) Phase I trial of an interleukin-2 receptor (IL-2R) fusion toxin (DAB_{486} IL-2) in hematologic malignancies expressing the IL-2 receptor. Blood 79:2547–2554

LeMaistre CF, Craig FE, Meneghetti C, McMullin B, Parker K, Reuben J, Boldt DH, Rosenblum M, Woodworth T (1993) Phase I trail of a 90-minute infusion of the fusion toxin DAB_{486} IL 2 in hematologic cancers. Cancer Res 53:3930–3934

Lemoine N, Hughes C, Barton C, Poulson R, Jeffery R, Kloppel G, HallP, Gullick W (1992) The epidermal growth factor receptor in human pancreatic cancer. J Pathol 166:7

Middlebrook JL, Dorland RB, Leppla SH (1978) Association of diphtheria toxin with Vero cells: demonstration of a receptor. J Biol Chem 253:7325–7330

Morris G, Dodd J (1990) Epidermal growth factor receptor mRNA levels in human prostatic tumors and cell lines. J Urol 143:1272

Morris RE, Gerstein AS, Bonventre PF, Saelinger CB (1985) Receptor-mediated entry of diphtheria toxin into monkey kidney (Vero) cells: electron microscopic evaluation. Infect Immun 50:721–727

Moya M, Dautry-Versat A, Goud B, Louvard D, Boquet P (1985) Inhibition of coated pit formation in Hep_2 cells blocks the cytotoxicity of diphtheria toxin but not that of ricin toxin. J Cell Biol 101:548–559

Murphy JR, Pappenheimer AM Jr, Tayart de Borms S (1974) Synthesis of diphtheria tox gene products in Escherichia coli extracts. Proc Natl Acad Sci USA 71:11–15

Murphy JR, Bishai W, Borowski M, Miyanohara A, Boyd J, Nagle S (1986) Genetic construction, expression, and melanoma-selective cytotoxicity of a diphtheria toxin α-melanocyte stimulating hormone fusion toxin. Proc Natl Acad Sci USA 83:8258–8262

Myers DA, Villemez CL (1988) Specific chemical cleavage of diphtheria toxin with hydroxyamine: purification and characterization of the modified proteins. J Biol Chem 263:17122–17127

Neal D, Mellon K (1992) Epidermal growth factor receptor and bladder cancer. Urol Int 48:365

Nicholson S, Halcrow P, Sainsbury J, Angus B, Chambers P, Farndon J, Harris A (1988) Epidermal growth factor receptor status associated with failure of primary endocrine therapy in elderly postmenopausal patients with breast cancer. Br J Cancer 58:810

Nickoloff BJ, Griffiths CEM (1990) Lymphocyte trafficking in psoriasis: a new perspective emphasizing the dermal dendrocyte with active dermal recruitment mediated via endothelial cells followed by intraepidermal T cell activation. J Invest Dermatol 95:35S–37S

Papini E, Sandoná D, Rappuoli R, Montecucco C (1988) On the membrane translocation of diphtheria toxin: at low pH the toxin induces ion channels in cells. EMBO J 7:3353–3359

Rolf JM, Eidels L (1993) Structure-function analyses of diphtheria toxin by use of monoclonal antibodies. Infect Immun 61:944–1003

Rosolen A, Nakanishi M, Poplack D, Cole D, Quinines R, Reaman G, Cotelingam J, Trepel J, Sausville E, Marti G, Neckers L, Colamonici O (1989) Expression of interleukin-2 receptor beta subunit in hematopoietic malignancies. Blood 73:1968–1972

Sandvig K, Olsnes S (1988) Diphtheria toxin-induced channels in Vero cells selective for monovalent cations. J Biol Chem 263:12352–12359

Schwartz G, Tepler I, Charette J, Kadin L, Parker K, Woodworth T, Schnipper L (1992) Complete response of a Hodgkin's lymphoma in a phase I trail of DAB$_{486}$ IL-2. Blood 79:175a

Shaw JP, Akiyoshi DE, Arrigo DA, Rhoad AE, Sullivan B, Thomas J, Genbauffe FS, Bacha P, Nichols JC (1991) Cytotoxic properties of DAB$_{486}$ EGF and DAB$_{389}$ EGF, epidermal growth factor (EGF) receptor-targeted fusion toxins. J Biol Chem 266:13449–13455

Sheibani K, Winberg C, van de Velde S, Blayney D, Rappaport H (1987) Distribution of lymphocytes with interleukin-2 receptors (TAC antigens) in reactive lymphoproliferative processes, Hodgkins disease, and non-Hodgkins lymphomas. An immunohistochemical study of 300 cases. Am J Pathol 127:27–37

Smith K, Fennelly J, Neal D, Hall R, Harris A (1989) Characterization and quantitation of epidermal growth factor receptors in invasive and superficial bladder tumors. Cancer Res 49:5810

Steele R, Kelly P, Ellul B, Ermin O (1990) Epidermal growth factor receptor expression in colorectal cancer. Br J Surg 77:1352

Strauchen J, Breakstone B (1987) IL-2 receptor expression in human lymphoid lesions. Am J Pathol 126:506–512

Takeshita T, Asao H, Ohtani K, Ishii N, Kumaki S, Tanaka N, Munakata H, Nakamura M, Sugamura K (1992) Cloning of the chain of the human IL-2 receptor. Science 257:379–382

Theodoulou M, Baselga J, Scher H, Dantis L, Trainor K, Mendelsohn J, Bacha P, Brandt-Sarif T, Osborne K (1995) Phase I dose escalation study of the safety, tolerability, and pharmacokinetics of DAB389EGF in patients with solid malignancies expressing EGF receptors. Proc ASCO 14:480

Uchida T, Gill DM, Pappenheimer AM Jr (1971) Mutation in the structural gene for diphtheria toxin carried by temperate phage β. Nature 233:8–11

Uchida T, Pappenheimer AM Jr, Greaney R (1973) Diphtheria toxin and related proteins: isolation and properties of mutant proteins serologically related to diphtheria toxin. J Biol Chem 248:3838–3844

Uchiyama T, Hori T, Tsudo M, Wano Y, Umadome H, Tamori S, Yodoi J, Maeda M, Sawami H, Uchino H (1985) Interleukin-2 receptor (Tac antigen) expressed on adult T cell leukemia cells. Clin Invest 76:446

Veale D, Ker N, Gibson G, Harris A (1989) Characterization of epidermal growth factor receptor in primary human non-small cell lung cancer. Cancer Res 49:1313

Vyse TJ, Todd JA (1996) Genetic analysis of autoimmune disease. Cell 85:311–318

Waldmann TA (1986) The structure, function, and expression of interleukin-2 receptors on normal and malignant T cells. Science 232:727–732

Waldmann TA (1990) The multichain interleukin-2 receptor. A target for immunotherapy in lymphoma, autoimmune disorders, and organ allografts. J Am Med Assoc 263:272–274

Walz G, Zanker B, Brand K, Swanlund D, Genbauffe F, Zeldis J, Murphy J, Strom T (1989) Sequential effects of interleukin-2/diphtheria toxin fusion protein on T cell activation. Proc Natl Acad Sci USA 86:9485–9488

Waters CA, Schimke P, Snider CE, Itoh K, Smith KA, Nichols JC, Strom TB, Murphy JR (1990) Interleukin-2 receptor targeted cytotoxicity: receptor binding requirements for entry of IL-2-toxin into cells. Eur J Immunol 20:785–791

Weidmann E, Sacchi M, Plaisance S, Heo D, Yasumura S, Lin W, Johnson J, Herberman R, Assarone B, Whiteside T (1992) Receptors for interleukin-2 on human squamous cell carcinoma cell lines and tumors in-situ. Cancer Res 52:5963–5970

Weinstein GD, Krueger JG (1993) An overview of psoriasis. In: Weinstein GD, Gottlieb AB (eds) Therapy of moderate-to-severe psoriasis. National Psoriasis Foundation, Portland, OR, pp 1–22

Wen Z, Tao X, Lakkis F, Kiyokawa T, Murphy JR (1991) Expression, purification, and α-melanocyte stimulating hormone receptor-specific toxicity of DAB-α-MSH fusion toxins. J Biol Chem 266:12289–12293

Williams D, Parker K, Bishai W, Borowski M, Genbauffe F, Strom TB, Murphy JR (1987) Diphtheriatoxin receptor binding domain substitution with interleukin-2: genetic construction and properties of a diphtheria toxin-related interleukin-2 fusion protein. Protein Engn 1:493–498

Williams D, Snider CE, Strom TB, Murphy JR (1990) Structure function analysis of IL-2 toxin (DAB$_{486}$ IL-2): fragment B sequences required for the delivery of fragment A to the cytosol of target cells. J Biol Chem 265:11885–11889

Clinical Trials with *Pseudomonas* Exotoxin Immunotoxins

L.H. Pai and I. Pastan

1	Background: Clinical Trial with First Generation Immunotoxin Using Native *Pseudomonas* Exotoxin	83
2	Second Generation *Pseudomonas* Exotoxin Immunotoxins:	86
2.1	Monoclonal Antibodies with Improved Selectivity	86
2.2	Recombinant Forms of *Pseudomonas* Exotoxin	87
3	Clinical Trial with Immunotoxin B3-LysPE38 (LMB-1)	87
4	Recombinant Single-Chain Immunotoxins with Improved Properties	90
4.1	Single-Chain Immunotoxin LMB-7	91
4.2	Single-Chain Immunotoxin Anti-Tac(Fv)-PE38	92
4.3	Recombinant Single-Chain Immunotoxin e23(Fv)-PE38	92
5	Other *Pseudomonas* Exotoxin Recombinant Toxins for Cancer Therapy	93
5.1	Intravesical Therapy of Transitional Cell Cancer with TP40 (TGFα-PE40)	93
6	Conclusion and Future Directions	94
	References	95

1 Background: Clinical Trial with First Generation Immunotoxin Using Native *Pseudomonas* Exotoxin

Pseudomonas exotoxin (PE) has been used to make immunotoxins for cancer therapy for more than a decade (FitzGerald et al. 1983). The function of PE is described in detail elsewhere in this book. In summary, PE is a 613 amino acid (66kDa) single-chain protein secreted by *Pseudomonas aeruginosa*. X-ray crystallography (Allured et al. 1986) and mutational studies (Gray et al. 1984; Hwang et al. 1987) have shown that PE is composed of three major structural and functional domains: an NH_2-terminal cell binding domain (domain Ia, composed of amino acids 1–252), a central translocation domain (domain II, amino acids 253–364), and a COOH-terminal domain (III, amino acids 399–613). The latter catalyzes the ADP-ribosylation and inactivation of elongation factor 2 and thereby

---

Laboratory of Molecular Biology, Division of Basic Sciences, National Cancer Institute, National Institutes of Health, Building 37, Room 4E16, 37 Convent Drive MSC 4255, Bethesda, MD 20892, USA

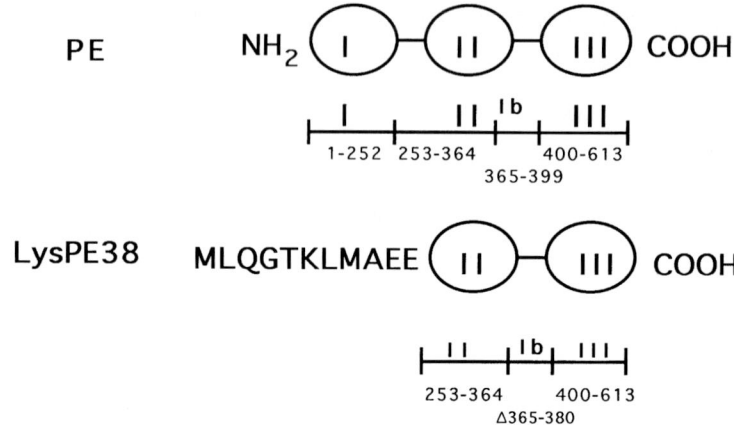

Fig. 1. *Pseudomonas* exotoxin (PE) and LysPE38

inhibits protein synthesis and leads to cell death. Domain III contain a COOH-terminal sequence (REDLK) that directs the endocytosed and processed toxin into the endoplasmic reticulum (see below). Substitution of REDLK with a KDEL sequence, which is known to retain newly synthesized proteins in the endoplasmic reticulum (SEETHARAM et al. 1991), results in a PE molecule that is more toxic to cells probably because it is more efficiently brought to the endoplasm reticulum where translocation seems to occur. Domain Ib is composed of amino acids 365–399 and has no known function; deletion of all of this domain results in no loss of activity (Fig. 1).

Cell killing is initiated when PE binds to a multifunctional, high molecular weight cell surface glycoprotein. This protein is the receptor for both α_2-macroglobulin and a low density lipoprotein (KOUNNAS et al. 1992). PE is then internalized by the pathway of receptor-mediated endocytosis (FITZGERALD et al. 1980). Upon reaching the endocytic compartment, the PE proenzyme is activated by a cleavage between amino acids 279 and 280 followed by reduction of a disulfide bond connecting amino acids 265–287. This generates a 37kDa fragment composed of a portion of domain II and all of domain III. The terminal lysine of PE is removed either by enzymes present in the plasma or within the cells. The 37kDa fragment is ultimately translocated to the cytosol, where it inactivates elongation factor 2 and produces cell death (IGLEWSKI and KABAT 1975).

The first immunotoxin made with PE utilized an anti-transferrin receptor monoclonal antibody as the targeting moiety. Anti-transferrin-PE receptor was shown to be active in tumors cells in vitro, with an IC_{50} of 0.1ng/ml (PIRKER et al. 1985). Because of the ubiquitous expression of the anti-transferrin receptor in eukaryotic cells, with the potential of multiple organ toxicity in patients, a decision was made not to proceed with its clinical development.

PE was also coupled to OVB3, a murine monoclonal antibody (IgG_{2b}) that reacts with all human ovarian cancers tested. The IC_{50} of OVB3-PE for inhibition of protein synthesis against the ovarian carcinoma cell line OVCAR-3 in vitro was

0.5ng/ml. When administered intraperitoneally, OVB3-PE was shown to prolong the life of nude mice bearing human ovarian tumor xenografts (WILLINGHAM et al. 1987; FITZGERALD et al. 1986).

A phase I study of OVB3-PE was conducted at the National Cancer Institute from November 1987 though November 1989 in patients with ovarian cancer limited to the peritoneal cavity (PAI et al. 1991a). Twenty three patients with refractory ovarian cancer were treated intraperitoneally with escalating doses (1, 2, 5 or 10μg/kg) of OVB3-PE in a fixed schedule (day 1, 4) or fixed dose (5μg/kg), escalating schedule (day 1, 4, 7 or day 1, 3, 5). All patients had histological confirmation of refractory invasive epithelial cancer of the ovary limited to the peritoneal cavity following platinum-based chemotherapy. The mean age was 53 years (39–68 years old).

The dose-limiting toxicity of OVB3-PE was encephalopathy at 5 and 10μg/kg. Dose-limiting central neurologic toxicity occurred in three patients. Two incidents of reversible encephalopathy occurred among five patients treated at the 10μg/kg dose level and were characterized by confusion, apraxia and dysarthria. Fatal neurotoxicity occurred in one patient after a third dose of OVB3-PE at 5μg/kg dose level. MRI in this patient revealed inflammatory abnormalities in the brainstem, cerebellum, deep nuclei and deep white matter. This toxicity necessitated immediate termination of the study. Other drug-related side effects included: grade 1–2 abdominal pain in 19 patients (83%) with no evidence of inflammatory or hemorrhagic peritonitis on the basis of peritoneal fluid cell counts, grade 1–2 nausea/vomiting, fever and grade 1 elevations of SGOT, SGPT or alkaline phosphatase.

Peritoneal fluid levels of OVB3-PE was measured and exceeded the in vitro IC_{50} at all doses tested. Immunotoxin remained detectable up to 72h after dosing and achieved levels > 100ng/ml at 5–10μg/kg dose levels.

Serum levels of OVB3-PE were detectable for 72h (peak 24h) following doses of 5 or 10μg/kg. At the dose level of 5μg/kg, 4–13.6ng/ml of OVB3-PE were detected 24h after each i.p. infusion. Serum levels remained constant and were still detected 72h after the first i.p. dose, but were negligible before the second dose at 96h. At the dose level of 10μg/kg, serum levels were detected at 24h after infusion, with a mean level of 19ng/ml range (7–40ng/ml). It was no longer detectable prior to the second dose (96h after infusion). OVB3-PE was not detected in the CSF obtained 48–72h after dosing from two patients with neurotoxicity. All patients developed antibodies against mouse immunoglobulins (HAMA) and to PE within 2–3 weeks of therapy. Domain II of PE appeared to be the most immunogenic portion of the PE molecule. No clinical antitumor responses were observed in this trial.

OVB3 reacts with an unknown antigen on the surface of several human adenocarcinomas. It also reacts with a small number of normal human tissues. However, it does not react with any monkey or rodent tissues. Based on antibody localization studies using frozen sections of normal human tissue, pancreatic and thyroid toxicity was anticipated. However, toxicities to these organs were not observed but, instead, neurocortical toxicity proved to be dose-limiting with abnormalities in the brainstem, cerebellum, deep nuclei and deep white matter.

In view of the unexpected clinical toxicity, immunohistochemical studies were performed in fresh samples from various portions of normal human brain. Weak immunoreactivity of OVB3 was detected with the molecular layer of the cerebellum, but not in the cerebellar granular layer, white matter, capillaries and cortical gray matter. Similar studies were performed in monkey brain tissue, which showed no reactivity to OVB3-PE. This explains the lack of neurologic symptoms in preclinical experiments performed in these primates. Although we were not able to detect the presence of OVB3-PE in the CSF, it is possible that small amounts of the immunotoxin not detectable by our assay (< 4ng/ml) may have entered the cerebrospinal space and damaged critical cells in the brain due to reactivity with monoclonal antibody OVB3. It is very unlikely that the neurotoxicity seen in these patients was due to free PE, since the thioether bond used for conjugation is known to be very stable. Thus, the neurotoxicity observed in this trial was most likely due to the specific reactivity of OVB3 with certain brain cells, which was not detected in the preclinical screening.

From this and other studies using ricin immunotoxins to target solid tumors, we conclude that immunotoxins are extremely active molecules that kill cells expressing the specific antigen on their surface. To prevent unanticipated clinical toxicity, antibodies selected for use in immunotoxins must be highly specific to tumor cells. If any cross-reactivity with normal human tissues is present, it would be desirable for the monoclonal antibody to react with the tissues of nonhuman primates (or other animals) to permit a very thorough preclinical evaluation of toxicity.

2 Second Generation *Pseudomonas* Exotoxin Immunotoxins

2.1 Monoclonal Antibodies with Improved Selectivity

Monoclonal antibody (MAb) B3 is an example of an antibody that reacts with many cancers and has better selectivity than OVB3. The hybridoma that produces MAb B3 (IgG$_{1k}$) was isolated from the spleen of a mouse immunized with MCF-7 (human breast carcinoma) cells (PASTAN et al. 1991). Biochemical analysis indicated that MAb B3 reacts with a carbohydrate antigen in the Le^y family that is present on many cell surface glycoproteins. These range in molecular weight from greater than 200,000kDa to less than 40,000kDa. Because many of these glycoproteins are internalized, they represent good targets for immunotoxin therapy.

A total of 382 tumors samples from patients with solid tumors have been screened for B3 reactivity by Dr. Mark Willingham at the University of South Carolina. Results are shown in Table 1. Using paraffin embedded tumor samples he found that 93% all adenocarcinomas of the colon react with MAb B3 and at least 75% of them react very strongly and homogeneously. Other gastrointestinal malignancies such as adenocarcinomas of the esophagus and stomach showed similar

Table 1. B3 Reactivity: immunohistochemical results (from 382 patients we have screened)

Primary Site	N	+B3	(%)
Colorectal	229	212	(93)
Breast	95	76	(80)
Esophagus/stomach	20	18	(90)
Pancreas/Bile duct	12	10	(83)
Lung	12	8	(66)
Ovary	8	4	(50)
Small Bowel	3	3	(100)
Bladder	4	2	(50)
Others[a]	10	0	(0)

[a] Salivary glands (2), prostate (2), sarcomas (2), skin (2), kidney (2)

strong reactivity in 90% of the samples tested. Some 80% of the breast carcinomas and 66% of adenocarcinomas of the lung express the B3 antigen. MAb B3 also reacts strongly with 50% of the mucinous adenocarcinomas of the ovary and transitional cell carcinoma of the bladder.

Peroxidase immunohistochemistry with frozen sections of normal tissues demonstrated that MAb B3 reacts with the glands of the stomach, the differentiated cell layer of the esophagus, and the epithelia of the trachea and bladder. Similar reactivity was found in cynomolgus monkeys and human tissues so that monkeys could be used for toxicology studies.

2.2 Recombinant Forms of *Pseudomonas* Exotoxin

When administered to animals, native PE causes acute liver necrosis due to the binding of domain Ia to hepatocytes. In order to decrease this nonspecific toxicity, domain Ia (amino acids 1–252) of PE was removed by recombinant DNA technology. The resulting molecule, PE40 was found to be 200-fold less toxic to mice than PE (KONDO et al. 1988). Deletion of amino acids 365–384 of domain Ib resulted in a smaller molecule, PE38, that retains full ADP-ribosylation activity and is also 200-fold less toxic to mice than native PE (KREITMAN et al. 1993). Figure 1 shows the schematic representation of PE and PE38.

Both PE40 and PE38 have been used to make second generation immunotoxins with less nonspecific liver toxicity. A peptide with a lysine residue was placed at the NH_2-terminal of PE38 to facilitate chemical coupling.

3 Clinical Trial with Immunotoxin B3(Lys)-PE38 (LMB-1)

LMB-1 B3(Lys)-PE38 is an immunotoxin in which MAb B3 is chemically coupled to LysPE38. In vitro, LMB-1 B3(Lys)-PE38 is very cytotoxic to several human carcinoma cell lines that express the B3 antigen on their surface, with IC_{50}s ranging from 1 to 10ng/ml (PAI et al. 1991b). In athymic mice, LMB-1 caused complete and lasting regressions of two human carcinomas (A431, an epidermoid carcinoma and MCF-7, a breast carcinoma) (PAI et al. 1992). Preclinical toxicity was assessed in cynomolgus monkeys because expression of the B3 antigen in normal monkeys is similar to that found in human tissue. The limiting toxicity in monkeys was found to be gastric mucosa necrosis and hemorrhage at the dose of 5mg/kg i.v. × three doses. Based on the immunohistochemical staining, this toxicity was predicted (PAI and PASTAN 1993).

A phase I trial of LMB-1 in cancer patients was conducted at the Medicine Branch, National Cancer Institute (PAI et al. 1996). Patients eligible for this study had a histologic diagnosis of a malignant solid tumor and had exhausted the standard therapeutic options for their disease, or had a malignant disease for which no established therapy exists. Tumor must express the B3 antigen on the surface of > 30% of the cells and they must not have preexisting neutralizing antibodies to LMB-1. Thirty eight patients with advanced solid tumors were enrolled in this study from July 1993 though December 1996. Sixteen patients were male and 22 patients were female, with a mean age of 47 (range 30–70). Twenty-six patients had colorectal cancer, eight breast cancer, one cancer of the esophagus, one cancer of the stomach, one ovarian cancer and one cancer of the ampulla of Vater. Patients received doses ranging from 10 to 100µg/kg (10, 15, 25, 30, 45, 70, 90 and 100µg/kg). Three to six patients were treated at each dose level. The starting dose was 100µg/kg, 1/30 of LD_{10} in mice (3.35mg/kg). Doses were subsequently reduced to 10µg/kg due to the occurrence of grade IV toxicity.

The major side effect of LMB-1 was found to be vascular leak syndrome, manifested by hypoalbuminemia, fluid retention and peripheral edema. At doses higher than 75µg/kg, transient postural hypotension and oliguria that did not require presser agents were observed in some patients. Pulmonary edema and severe hypotension occurred in one patient who received 100µg/kg. Other less frequent and well-tolerated side effects include "flu-like" symptoms, fever, malaise, skin rash, headache and nonspecific EKG changes. All drug-related side effects occurred during the week of therapy and resolved within 2 weeks. Although normal tissues such as mucosal surface of the stomach, trachea and bladder, exocrine glands of the pancreas and the colloid of the thyroid gland do express Le^y antigen[1], no drug related side effects were observed. The maximum tolerated dose of LMB-1 was defined as 75µg/kg every other day × three doses.

Antitumor activity was observed in five patients, 18 patients had stable disease, 15 patients progressed. A complete remission lasting 2 months was observed in a 40 year old female with metastatic breast cancer to the supraclavicular lymph nodes. This patient received two cycles of LMB-1 at 15µg/kg. Shrinkage of supraclavicular nodes was observed 5–7 days after the first dose of LMB-1. A greater than 75% tumor reduction was observed in a 50 year old male with extensive metastatic colon cancer to the abdomen and supraclavicular lymph nodes. Tumor shrinkage was observed after one single dose of LMB-1 at 90µg/kg (Fig. 2). Because this patient did not developed antibodies, he received three additional cycles

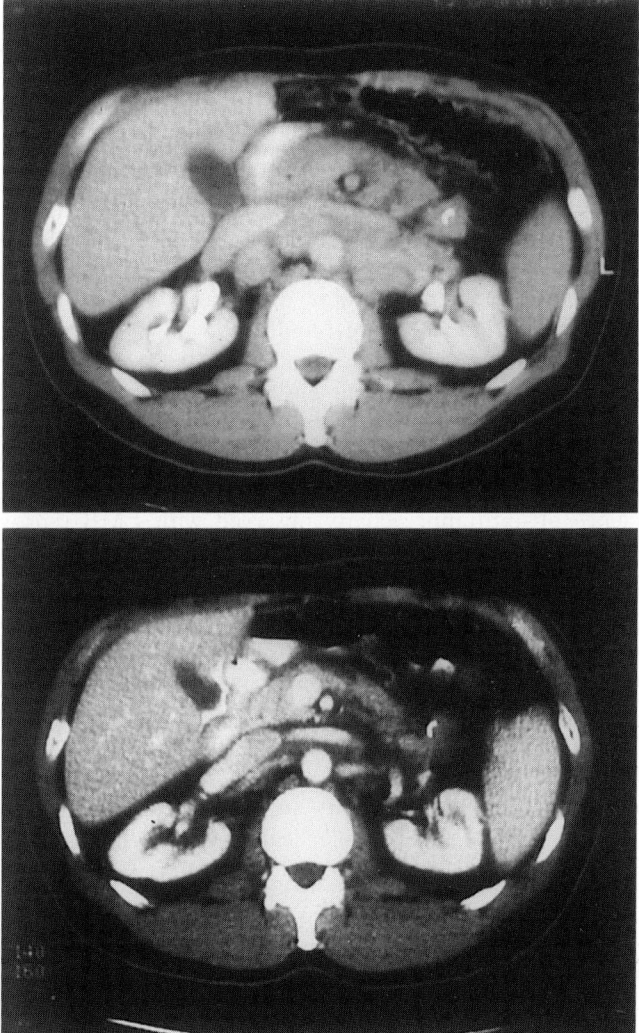

Fig. 2. Computerized tomography scan of a 50 year old male with colon cancer treated with LMB-1. *Upper scan*: extensive retroperitoneal adenopathy prior to therapy. *Lower scan*: after two cycles of LMB-1 there is marked tumor shrinkage

of LMB-1 at 50% (45µg/kg) dose reduction. Dose was reduced due to grade 3 toxicity after cycle 1. CT scan of the abdomen show that the tumor continued to decrease in size after each cycle. This patient was followed without evidence of disease progression for > 6 months. Prior to therapy, the patient complained of chronic diarrhea and abdominal pain which required therapy with acetaminophen plus codeine. Symptoms resolved completely after treatment. Biological responses (< 50% decrease in tumor size and/or tumor shrinkage lasting less than a month) were observed in three additional patients who received 10, 75 and 90µg/kg. One colon cancer patient had shrinkage of pulmonary nodules lasting for up to 9 months. Minor responses were observed in two other patients, one colon cancer patient with transient decrease of an inguinal mass lasting for < 4 weeks and a breast cancer patient with adrenal metastasis who had < 50% tumor reduction lasting 2 months. Stable patients that could not be retreated due to presence of antibodies against LMB-1 were followed until disease progression. The median time to disease progression was 3 months (range 1–9 months).

Immunogenicity of LMB-1 was assessed by using ELISA and serum neutralization assays. Some 90% (33/38) of the patients developed neutralizing antibodies against LMB-1 3 weeks after one cycle of treatment. Three patients received two cycles of LMB-1 (10, 15, 60µg/kg) and one patient received four cycles (90/45µg/kg). ELISA assay indicated that all patients (38/38) developed antibody titers against PE38 and 33 of 38 had antibody titers against MAb B3. These findings indicate that, although all patients formed antibodies against the toxin moiety, these antibodies have no neutralizing effect against the LMB-1 in 15% of the cases.

The evidence of antitumor activity observed with LMB-1 proves that it is possible to target epithelial malignancies in humans. Although immunotoxin therapy has been shown to be active in hematologic malignancies, this is the first time that objective antitumor activity against metastatic colon and breast cancers has been documented. At the maximum tolerated dose, side effects of LMB-1 were well-tolerated and transient. The major side effect, vascular leak syndrome, is secondary to targeting of LMB-1 to antigen-positive endothelial cells. Phase II studies using LMB-1 are presently being planned to target patients with epithelial tumors with minimal residual disease. Concomitant use of LMB-1 with high dose steroids is presently being investigated in an attempt to suppress neutralizing antibody formation and ameliorate vascular leak syndrome.

4 Recombinant Single-Chain Immunotoxins with Improved Properties

The third generation PE-containing immunotoxins are composed of the variable regions of the light and heavy chains of an antibody directly fused to truncated forms of PE (CHAUDHARY et al. 1989, 1990). Single-chain immunotoxins have several advantages over chemical conjugates such as OVB3-PE and LMB-1 (B3-LysPE38). They are more active when compared to chemical conjugates, they are more homogeneous, less costly to produce and less immunogenic. However their most important property is that due to their smaller size compared to chemical conjugates (66kDa × 200kDa) they should have better tumor penetration.

Antibodies are large molecules in which the antigen recognition site contained in the light and heavy chain variable domains is connected to a large constant region that has several different effector functions. The smallest antibody fragment that can bind antigen with high affinity is the Fv region (fragment variable), which consists of two chains each about 110 amino acids in length. The two chains are not naturally linked together and therefore usually form unstable complexes, but these can be stabilized by connecting them together with a linking peptide of about 15 amino acids in length. The product is a single-chain antigen-binding protein or single-chain antibody. These small molecules can have high affinity for antigen, and have been used to target cells by genetically fusing PE40 or PE38 to their carboxyl end. Several single-chain immunotoxins have been made with PE40 and PE38 and are presently or undergoing clinical investigation or are in late phases of preclinical development (Table 2).

4.1 Single-Chain Immunotoxin LMB-7

LMB-7 (B3Fv-PE38) is the recombinant single-chain counterpart of LMB-1 (chemical conjugate B3-LysPE38). The cloned genes encoding the heavy and light chain Fv regions of MAb B3 were fused to the gene encoding PE38 to generate the single-chain immunotoxin B3(Fv)-PE38, also termed LMB-7 (BRINKMANN et al. 1991). LMB-7 is very cytotoxic to carcinoma cell lines that express the B3 antigen and causes complete regressions of a human breast carcinoma (MCF-7) and an epidermoid carcinoma (A431) growing in immunodeficient mice. Complete remission of tumors was achieved with 0.075mg/kg given every other day × three doses and very significant antitumor effects occurred at lower doses. These findings indicate that LMB-7 is more active than LMB-1, even taking the differences in molecular weight into consideration. Figure 3 shows a schematic figure of LMB-1 and LMB-7 emphasizing their major differences. A clinical trial using LMB-7 in patients with solid tumors is presently being conducted at the Medicine Branch, National Cancer Institute. Results of this trial should be available within a year.

Table 2. *Pseudomonas* exotoxin immunotoxins for cancer therapy

Immunotoxin	Target antigen	Disease	Major toxicity	Reference
OVB3-PE	?	Ovarian cancer (i.p.)	Encephalopathy	FITZGERALD et al. 1986
TP40	EGFR	Bladder cancer (intravesical)	None	GOLDBERG et al. 1995
LMB-1 (B3-LysPE38)	Le^y	Adenocarcinomas	Vascular leak syndrome	PAI et al. 1996
LMB-2 (Anti-Tac-Fv PE38)	Interleukin-2 receptor (p55)	Lymphomas	Ongoing	
LMB-7 (B3Fv-PE38)	Le^y	Adenocarcinomas	Ongoing	
Preclinical testing				
e23-(Fv)-PE38	Erb-2	Breast, gastric, lung cancer	–	BATRA et al. 1992; REITER et al. 1994
B3(dsFv)-PE38	Le^y	Adenocarcinomas	–	
RFB4(Fv)-PE38	CD22	Lymphoma	–	

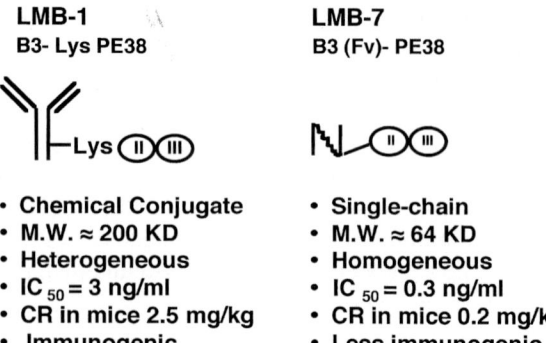

Fig. 3. Schematic representation of immunotoxins LMB-1 and LMB-7 and their preclinical characteristics

4.2 Single-Chain Immunotoxin Anti-Tac(Fv)-PE38

The first single-chain immunotoxin constructed employed anti-Tac, an antibody to the p55 subunit of the human interleukin (IL)-2 receptor (CHAUDHARY et al. 1990). The Fv regions of the anti-Tac antibody were genetically fused to PE40. Anti-Tac(Fv)-PE40 and derivatives are very cytotoxic to IL2 receptor-bearing human cell lines and peripheral blood malignant cells from patients with adult T cell leukemia (KREITMAN et al. 1990). They also cause complete tumor regressions in nude mice bearing tumors that overexpress the IL2 receptor (KREITMAN et al. 1994). Because anti-Tac(Fv)PE38 was found to be active against a variety of leukemia and lymphoma cell lines, a phase I clinical trial using anti-Tac(Fv)PE38 was opened for patient accrual late in 1996 and is presently being conducted at National Cancer Institute by Dr. Robert Kreitman.

4.3 Recombinant Single-Chain Immunotoxin e23(Fv)-PE38

To exploit the overexpression of erbB-2 in many human cancers (breast, stomach, lung and ovary), a single-chain immunotoxin was made using MAb e23 that reacts with erbB-2. This single-chain immunotoxin is specifically cytotoxic to cells expressing erbB-2 and causes regression of the human gastric cancer cells (N87) and epidermoid carcinoma cells growing as tumors in immunodeficient mice (BATRA et al. 1992). The Fv fragment of MAb e23 is unstable and has a diminished affinity compared to the original antibody. These differences were overcome by stabilizing the Fv with a disulfide bound to make e23(dsFv)PE38 (REITER et al. 1994). This and several other recombinant immunotoxins are undergoing preclinical development and should be available for clinical testing in cancer patients within the next few years.

5 Other *Pseudomonas* Exotoxin Recombinant Toxins for Cancer Therapy

Several chimeric toxins have been made by fusing a portion of the PE gene to cDNAs encoding growth factors or cytokines. These include transforming growth factor (TGF)-α (CHAUDHARY et al. 1987), insulin-like growth factor (IGF)-1 (PRIOR et al. 1991), acidic and basic fibroblast growth factor (FGF) (SIEGALL et al. 1991), IL2 (LORBERBOUM-GALSKI et al. 1988), IL4 (DEBINSKI et al. 1993) and IL6 (SIEGALL et al. 1990). These oncotoxins are designed to target specific tumor cells that overexpress these receptors and are in different stages of preclinical and clinical development.

5.1 Intravesical Therapy of Transitional Cell Cancer with TP40 (TGFα-PE40)

The DNA encoding TGFα has been fused to PE40 to form the chimeric toxin TGFα-PE40 (CHAUDHARY et al. 1987), which specifically kills cells that overexpress EGF receptor. When given by i.p. infusion to immunodeficient mice bearing subcutaneous tumors which express EGF receptors, it caused partial regressions (PAI et al. 1991c). However, because several normal organs, and particularly the liver, express the EGF receptor (EGFR), the therapeutic window for TGFα-PE40 is narrow when delivered systemically. To circumvent liver toxicity, this agent has been used for the regional therapy of superficial bladder cancer in patients.

Transitional cell cancer of the bladder is known to overexpress EGFRs and tumors with a high density of EGFR have been shown to have a poorer clinical outcome than tumors with fewer receptors (NEAL et al. 1990). A phase I trial using a genetically modified form of TGFα-PE40, termed TP40 (HEIMBROOK et al. 1990), was carried out in patients with superficial bladder cancer. Forty-three patients were entered into this study (GOLDBERG et al. 1995). Therapy was given weekly × 6 by intravesical administration at doses ranging from 0.15mg to 9.6mg. No toxicities were observed in this study. Eleven patients had evaluable Ta or T1 lesions, 19 had resected Ta or T1 lesions, seven had carcinoma in situ only and six patients had mixed carcinoma in situ (CIS) and stage Ta/T1 disease. Eighteen of 18 tumor samples tested were positive for EGFR. One complete remission occurred in a patient with CIS, five of seven (70%) of the patients with CIS were found to have visual resolution of the lesions during follow-up cystoscopy. Two out of five patients continued to have positive cytology during follow-up, one patient had resolution of bladder lesions, but CIS persisted in the prostatic urethra; one patient recurred with Ta lesions and one patient remained in complete remission after more than 5 months. This last patient had a history of multiple panurothelial Ta and CIS lesions that failed BCG treatment and had multiple recurrences after surgical resections. Prior to receiving TP40, cystoscopy revealed multiple areas of CIS in the bladder. The patient received six doses of TP40 at 9.6mg/dose without complications, side effects or toxicity. Follow-up cystoscopies revealed a normal bladder and the urinary cytology has remained negative 5 months after treatment. None of the patients in this trial developed antibodies against TP40.

The evidence of biological activity of TP40 in CIS patients in this phase I study is encouraging. Further trials using prolonged bladder irrigation, daily intravesical administrations or other schemes of delivery might help improve the efficacy of this agent for patients with superficial bladder cancer.

6 Conclusions and Future Directions

The most important conclusion from our studies is that it is possible to obtain regression of solid tumors in patients treated with immunotoxins containing *Pseudomonas* exotoxin A. It is particularly striking that responses were observed in patients with colon cancer, because colon cancer is a very common disease and colon cancers are resistant to current therapies. Moreover, responses were also observed in breast cancer. Based on these phase I studies, phase II trials with LMB-1 will be carried out targeting specific cancers in patients with minimal residual disease following surgery or other therapies.

An unexpected side effect of LMB-1 was vascular leak syndrome. Our evidence indicates that vascular leak syndrome is due to a small amount of antigen on endothelial cells combined with the long half-life of LMB-1 in the circulation, so that the endothelial cells are exposed to high concentrations of LMB-1 for a prolonged period (KUAN et al. 1995). We have recently began trials with a small recombinant immunotoxin (LMB-7) containing the Fv portion of monoclonal antibody B3. These small molecules (molecular weight 64,000) rapidly leave the circulation and should produce less vascular leak syndrome. A second and more stable recombinant immunotoxin, LMB-9, also directed at Le^y, will enter trials sometime in 1997. These single-chain immunotoxins are also less immunogenic than LMB-1. We plan try to combine these immunotoxins with immunosuppressive drugs so that repeated cycles can be given.

A major problem with recombinant immunotoxin therapy is the specificity of the antibody. MAb B3 and antibodies to erb2 are known to react with essential normal tissues so that there is a small window between response and targeted side effects. It would be desirable to target antigens that are not present on normal cells. Two approaches to this problem have been developed. One is to target mutant molecules such as mutant receptors on the surface of cancer cells. A recombinant immunotoxin that binds only to a mutant form of the EGFR has recently been produced (LORIMER et al. 1996). The second is to target peptide MHC-peptide complexes present on the surface of tumor cells. We have recently made an immunotoxin that recognizes a peptide-MHC complex in which the peptide is derived from a virus. Immunotoxins against this complex are very active in killing target cells (REITER et al. 1997). Our plan is to try and generate monoclonal antibodies that recognize MHC-peptide complexes in which the peptides are derived from intracellular antigens such as mutant p53 or mutant ras. These mutant peptides are very attractive candidates for future immunotherapy.

References

Allured VS, Collier RJ, Carroll SF, McKay DB (1986) Structure of exotoxin A of Pseudomonas aeruginosa at 3.0 Angstrom resolution. Proc Natl Acad Sci USA 83:1320–1324
Batra JK, Kasprzyk PG, Bird RE, Pastan I, King CR (1992) Recombinant anti-erbB2 immunotoxins containing Pseudomonas exotoxin. Proc Natl Acad Sci USA 89:5867–5871
Brinkmann U, Pai LH, FitzGerald DJ, Pastan I (1991) B3(Fv)-PE38KDEL, a single-chain immunotoxin that causes complete regression of a human carcinoma in mice. Proc Natl Acad Sci USA 88:8616–8620
Chaudhary VK, FitzGerald DJ, Adhya S, Pastan I (1987) Activity of a recombinant fusion protein between transforming growth factor type α and Pseudomonas toxin. Proc Natl Acad Sci USA 84:4538–4542
Chaudhary VK, Queen C, Junghans RP, Waldmann TA, FitzGerald DJ, Pastan I (1989) A recombinant immunotoxin consisting of two antibody variable domains fused to Pseudomonas exotoxin. Nature 339:394–397
Chaudhary VK, Batra JK, Gallo M, Willingham MC, Pastan I (1990) A rapid method of cloning functional variable region antibody genes in E. coli as single-chain immunotoxins. Proc Natl Acad Sci USA 87:1066–1070
Debinski W, Puri RK, Kreitman RJ, Pastan I (1993) A wide range of human cancer express IL4 receptor that can be targeted with chimeric toxin composed of IL4 and Pseudomonas exotoxin. J Biol Chem 268:14065–14070
FitzGerald DJ, Morris RE, Saelinger CB (1980) Receptor-mediated internalization of Pseudomonas toxin by mouse fibroblasts. Cell 21:867–873
FitzGerald DJ, Trowbridge IS, Pastan I, Willingham MC (1983) Enhancement of toxicity of antitransferrin receptor antibody-Pseudomonas exotoxin conjugates by adenovirus. Proc Natl Acad Sci USA 80:4134–4138
FitzGerald DJ, Willingham MC, Pastan I (1986) Antitumor effects of an immunotoxin made with Pseudomonas exotoxin in a nude mouse model of human ovarian cancer. Proc Natl Acad Sci USA 83:6627–6630
Goldberg MR, Heimbrook DC, Russo P, Sarosdy MF, Greenberg RE, Giantonio BJ, Linehan WM, Walther M, Fisher HAG, Messing E, Crawford ED, Oliff AI, Pastan I (1995) Phase I clinical study of the recombinant oncotoxin TP40 in superficial bladder cancer. Clin Cancer Res 1:57–61
Gray GL, Smith DH, Baldridge JS, Harkins RN, Vasil ML, Chen EY, Heyneker HL (1984) Cloning, nucleotide sequence and expression in Escherichia coli of the exotoxin A structural gene of Pseudomonas aeruginosa. Proc Natl Acad Sci USA 8:2645–2649
Heimbrook DC, Stirdivant SM, Ahern JD, Balishin NL, Patrick DR, Edwards GM (1990) Transforming growth factor-α-Pseudomonas exotoxin fusion protein prolongs survival of nude mice bearing tumor xenografts. Proc Natl Acad Sci USA 87:4697–4701
Hwang J, FitzGerald DJ, Adhya S, Pastan I (1987) Functional domains of Pseudomonas exotoxin identified by deletion analysis of the gene expressed in E. coli. Cell 48:129–136
Iglewski BH, Kabat D (1975) NAD-dependent inhibition of protein synthesis by Pseudomonas aeruginosa toxin. Proc Natl Acad Sci USA 72:2284–2288
Kondo T, FitzGerald D, Chaudhary VK, Adhya S, Pastan I (1988) Activity of immunotoxins constructed with modified Pseudomonas exotoxin A lacking the cell recognition domain. J Biol Chem 263:9470–9475
Kounnas MZ, Morris RE, Thompson MR, FitzGerald DJ, Strickland DK, Saelinger CB (1992) The α_2-macroglobulin receptor/low density lipoprotein receptor-related protein binds and internalizes Pseudomonas exotoxin A. J Biol Chem 267:12420–12423
Kreitman RJ, Chaudhary VK, Waldmann T, Willingham MC, FitzGerald DJ, Pastan I (1990) The recombinant immunotoxin anti-Tac(Fv)-PE40 is cytotoxic toward peripheral blood malignant cells from patients with adult T-cell leukemia. Proc Natl Acad Sci USA 87:8291–8295

Kreitman RJ, Batra JK, Seetharam S, Chaudhary VK, FitzGerald DJ, Pastan I (1993) Single-chain immunotoxin fusions between anti-Tac and Pseudomonas exotoxin: relative importance of the two toxin disulfide bonds. Bioconj Chem 4:112–120

Kreitman RJ, Bailon P, Chaudhary VK, FitzGerald DJ, Pastan I (1994) Recombinant immunotoxin containing anti-Tac(Fv) and derivatives of PE produce complete regression in nude mice of an interleukin-2-receptor expressing human carcinoma. Blood 83:426–434

Kuan C-T, Pai LH, Pastan I (1995) Immunotoxins containing Pseudomonas exotoxin targeting Le^Y damage human endothelial cells in an antibody specific mode: relevance to vascular leak syndrome. Clin Cancer Res 1:1589–1594

Lorberboum-Galski H, FitzGerald D, Chaudhary V, Adhya S, Pastan I (1988) Cytotoxic activity of an interleukin 2-Pseudomonas exotoxin chimeric protein produced in E. coli. Proc Natl Acad Sci USA 85:1922–1926

Lorimer IAJ, Keppler-Hafkemeyer A, Beers R, Pegram C, Bigner D, Pastan I (1996) Recombinant immunotoxins specific for a mutant epidermal growth factor receptor: targeting with a single chain antibody variable domain isolated by phase display. Proc Natl Acad Sci USA 93:14815–14820

Neal DE, Sharples L, Smith K, Fennelly J, Hall RR, Harris AL (1990) The epidermal growth factor receptor and the prognosis of bladder cancer. Cancer 65:1619–1625

Pai LH, Pastan I (1993) Immunotoxin therapy for cancer. JAMA 269:78–81

Pai LH, Bookman MA, Ozols RJ, Young RC, Smith JW II, Longo DL, Gould B, Frankel A, McClay EF, Howell S, Reed E, Willingham MC, FitzGerald DJ, Pastan I (1991a) Clinical evaluation of intraperitoneal Pseudomonas exotoxin immunoconjugate OVB3-PE in patients with ovarian cancer. J Clin Oncol 9:2095–2103

Pai LH, FitzGerald DJ, Willingham MC, Pastan I (1991b) Antitumor activities of immunotoxins made of monoclonal antibody B3 and various forms of Pseudomonas exotoxin. Proc Natl Acad Sci USA 88:3358–3362

Pai LH, Gallo MG, FitzGerald DJ, Pastan I (1991c) Anti-tumor activity of a transforming growth factor α-Pseudomonas exotoxin fusion protein (TGFα-PE40). Cancer Res 51:2808–2812

Pai LH, Batra JK, FitzGerald DJ, Willingham MC, Pastan I (1992) Anti-tumor effects of B3-PE and B3-LysPE40 in a nude mouse model of human breast cancer and the evaluation of B3-PE toxicity in monkeys. Cancer Res 52:3189–3193

Pai LH, Wittes R, Setser A, Willingham MC, Pastan I (1996) Treatment of advanced solid tumors with immunotoxin LMB-1: an antibody linked to Pseudomonas exotoxin. Nature Med 3:350–353

Pastan I, Lovelace ET, Gallo MG, Rutherford AV, Magnani JL, Willingham MC (1991) Characterization of monoclonal antibodies B1 and B3 that react with mucinous adenocarcinomas. Cancer Res 51:3781–3787

Pirker R, FitzGerald DJP, Hamilton TC, Ozols RF, Willingham MC, Pastan I (1985) Anti-transferrin-receptor antibody linked to Pseudomonas exotoxin as a model immunotoxin in human ovarian carcinoma cell lines. Cancer Res 45:751–757

Prior TI, Helman LJ, FitzGerald DJ, Pastan I (1991) Cytotoxic activity of a recombinant fusion protein between insulin-like growth factor I and Pseudomonas exotoxin. Cancer Res 51:174–180

Reiter Y, Brinkmann U, Jung SH, Lee B, Kasprzyk PG, King CR, Pastan I (1994) Improved binding and antitumor activity of a recombinant anti-erbB2 immunotoxin by disulfide stabilization of the Fv fragment. J Biol Chem 269:18327–18331

Reiter Y, DiCarlo A, Guffer L, Engberg J, Pastan I (1997) Peptide-specific killing of antigen-presenting cells by a recombinant antibody-toxin fusion protein targeted to MHC/peptide class I complexes with T-cells receptor-like specificity. Proc Natl Acad Sci USA 94:4631–4636

Seetharam S, Chaudhary VT, FitzGerald D, Pastan I (1991) Increased cytotoxic activity of Pseudomonas exotoxin and the chimeric toxins ending in kDaEL. J Biol Chem 266:17376–17381

Siegall CB, Schwab G, Nordan RP, FitzGerald DJ, Pastan I (1990) Expression of the interleukin 6 receptor and interleukin 6 in prostate carcinoma cells. Cancer Res 50:7786–7788

Siegall CB, Epstein S, Speir E, Hla T, Forough R, Maciag T, FitzGerald D, Pastan I (1991) Cytotoxic activity of chimeric proteins composed of acidic fibroblast growth factor and Pseudomonas exotoxin on a variety of cell types. FASEB J 5:2843–2849

Willingham MC, FitzGerald D, Pastan I (1987) Pseudomonas exotoxin coupled to a monoclonal antibody against ovarian cancer inhibits the growth of human ovarian cancer cells in a mouse model. Proc Natl Acad Sci USA 84:2474–2478

Immunotoxins for Brain Tumor Therapy

E.H. Oldfield and R.J. Youle

1	Immunotoxins from the Diphtheria Toxin Mutant CRM107	97
2	The Transferrin Receptor as a Tumor Antigen	98
3	The Blood-Brain Barrier and Its Importance in Brain Tumors	99
4	Leptomeningeal Cancer	101
4.1	Preclinical Pharmacokinetics of Immunotoxins After Intrathecal Delivery	101
4.2	Preclinical Toxicity and Efficacy of Intrathecal Immunotoxin Administration/Antitumor Activity	101
4.3	Clinical Investigation	103
5	Parenchymal Tumor	106
5.1	Pharmacokinetics of Convection-Enhanced Drug Delivery	106
5.2	Preclinical Toxicity/Antitumor Activity	108
5.3	Clinical Trial	109
References		113

1 Immunotoxins from the Diphtheria Toxin Mutant CRM107

Cancer cells can be specifically killed by a class of therapeutic molecules called immunotoxins that combine the potent toxicity of natural plant and bacterial proteins with the tumor-specific binding capacity of monoclonal antibodies. Toxins such as ricin and diphtheria toxin have been linked to new cell surface binding moieties in order to target tumor cells for destruction. To the extent that tumor cells have cell surface receptors that distinguish them from normal and essential cells, immunotoxins can be considered as potential reagents for cancer therapy. Tumor cell specific ligands, such as growth factors or monoclonal antibodies, can be linked to protein toxins by random chemical modification of lysine or sulfhydral residues (Vitetta et al. 1987) or by fusion of the new protein domains at the COOH- or NH_2-terminal of the protein by molecular biology techniques (Pastan et al. 1986).

One of the most potent and specific immunotoxins generated to date expresses a cell-type-specificity of 200,000 fold between target and nontarget cells (Youle 1991).

Surgical Neurology Branch, National Institute of Neurological Disorders and Stroke, 10 Center Drive, Room 5D37, Bethesda, MD 20892, USA

The toxin, CRM107, is a single point mutant of diphtheria toxin initially isolated by random point mutagenesis and screening for nontoxic variants of diphtheria toxin (LAIRD and GROMAN 1976). Sequencing of CRM107 identified a single point mutation, serine to phenylalanine, at amino acid 525 (NICHOLLS et al. 1993). The point mutation inactivated the toxin binding activity and toxicity 10,000-fold (GREENFIELD et al. 1987). However, the translocation activity in the B-chain and the enzymatic activity were intact and resulted in fully potent immunotoxins upon coupling the mutant to monoclonal antibodies (GREENFIELD et al. 1987; JOHNSON et al. 1988). Thus, due to the large decrease in nonspecific toxicity due to the point mutation, the therapeutic window of the immunotoxin was greatly increased.

Ricin, a plant toxin, has also been linked to monoclonal antibodies to generate immunotoxins. Ricin A-chain linked to monoclonal antibodies to the transferrin receptor, for example, are extremely specific for target cells, although their potency has some interesting and marked differences compared to CRM107 linked to the same monoclonal antibodies (SUNG et al. 1991). It is important to determine the extent of cell type selectivity, the kinetics of cell killing and the log kill potential of different immunotoxins to assess clinical potential.

Thus, immunotoxins can be engineered to display extremely potent and specific toxicity in vitro. However, immunotoxin utility in clinical trials has been less successful due to three continuing problems. First, ideal tumor-specific antigens are found only in certain exceptional types of cancer (i.e., idiotype antigens on B cell leukemias). For brain tumor therapy a number of candidate tumor-associated receptors have been identified such as the epidermal growth factor, platelet derived growth factor, and interleukin (IL)-4 receptors. However, these antigens are present only on a subset of total patients and only a limited percentage of tumor cells in vivo may express them. Second, access of large proteins to tumor cells is limited for systemic tumors and is even more constrained for brain tumors by the blood-brain barrier. Lastly, immunogenicity of foreign toxin molecules has limited the delivery of an effective course of immunotoxin therapy.

2 The Transferrin Receptor as a Tumor Antigen

The degree to which tumor cells express entirely novel antigens is unknown. We have explored the potential of the transferrin receptor for therapy of brain tumors for a number of reasons. The transferrin receptor was originally identified as a tumor-associated antigen (TROWBRIDGE et al. 1982). Its level of expression is increased in a number of cancers as well as on rapidly growing tissues, apparently due to the increased iron requirements of dividing cells (GATTER et al. 1983). Within the CNS, normal astrocytes and neurons have undetectable levels of transferrin receptor expressed on their surface whereas several types of gliomas express quite high transferrin receptor levels (JOHNSON et al. 1989; MARTELL et al. 1993; RECHT et al. 1990; ZOVICKIAN et al. 1987). However, brain capillary endothelial cells also express transferrin receptors. Brain microvessels have three- to fivefold higher transferrin receptor levels than normal cortex (KALARIA et al. 1992). The transferrin receptor present on brain capillary endothelial cells appears to primarily face the lumen of the capillary (JEFFRIES et al. 1984) to mediate transcapillary transport of iron (SHIN et al. 1995). The sensitivity of normal brain to anti-transferrin receptor immunotoxins is about 3000 times lower than the sensitivity of numerous glioma cell lines in vitro suggesting that a therapeutic window may exist in vivo. The apparent advantages of the transferrin receptor as a tumor target are the wide variety of tumor types sensitive to anti-transferrin receptor immunotoxins; the requirement of iron (and thus the transferrin receptor) for tumor cell growth (indicating that tumor cell heterogeneity for antigen expression will be lower in the case of transferrin receptor than for other receptors not essentially linked to malignancy) and the extensive understanding of the distribution and physiological role of the native transferrin receptor, which has permitted thorough toxicity testing of immunotoxins targeted to animal transferrin (MURASZKO et al. 1993).

3 The Blood-Brain Barrier and Its Importance in Brain Tumors

Clinical trials to identify effective chemotherapeutic regimens for primary malignant brain tumors in adults over the past three decades generally have been disappointing. Reduced drug exposure of the tumors because of the presence of the blood-brain barrier (BBB) underlies at least some of the limitation of clinical efficacy.

The BBB limits the transfer of water-soluble substances from the blood to the brain, providing protection of the brain from fluctuations in the blood concentration of various circulating hydrophilic molecules. Although in malignant brain tumors the BBB is often altered (the endothelial cells of tumor vessels lose the intercellular tight junctions that are characteristic of CNS vessels), it retains some of its capacity to retard entry of water-soluble substances into the tumor. This reduced permeability of tumors in the brain is one of the reasons that patients with brain metastases often have progression of CNS tumors while tumor response to systemic chemotherapy is occurring at the primary site or at other sites outside the CNS. Moreover, in the most common types of primary brain tumors malignant glioma cells extend several centimeters from the contrast-enhancing regions seen on MRI, and the intact BBB at these distant sites limits exposure of the infiltrating malignant cells to most forms of systemic chemotherapy (BERGSTROM et al. 1983; EARNEST et al. 1988).

In efforts to increase drug delivery to cerebral tumors a variety of approaches have been examined, including the use of lipophilic drugs (FISHMAN and CHAN 1990), disruption of the BBB by intraarterial administration of hyperosmolar solutions such as mannitol (RAPOPORT et al. 1972), designing drugs with specific affinity to transmembrane carrier mechanisms (PARDRIDGE 1990), implantation of biodegradable polymers of chemotherapy (BREM et al. 1995), and continuous infusion of the drug into the brain (BOBO et al. 1994; MORRISON et al. 1994).

For the approaches that use intravascular delivery of the agent additional limitations arise, hindrances that are particularly relevant for some of the newer classes of antitumor agents, such as immunotoxins. These limitations include the systemic toxicity (hepatic damage, vascular leak syndrome) associated with the general exposure that occurs with intravenous or intraarterial injection of immunotoxins. They also include additional pharmacological barriers to distribution of immunotoxins to solid tumors. Solid tumors have elevated interstitial pressure relative to the interstitial pressure of surrounding normal tissues and in relation to capillary pressure (BOUCHER et al. 1990), poor perfusion of tumor vasculature (SEVICK and JAIN 1989), and binding effects (SUNG et al. 1993) all of which limit penetration of the immunotoxin into the tumor interstitium. Further, studies examining the spatial distribution of tumor-targeting immunotoxins in experimental tumors (after systemic administration) show tumor-specific binding occurring in a heterogeneous, punctate dispersion within the tumor (SUNG et al. 1993).

However, until drug design eliminates the toxicities associated with systemic exposure and until the development of immunity after exposure to foreign protein toxins has been reduced, there are also certain advantages of targeting tumors of the CNS. In most patients with primary brain tumors local and regional tumor growth cause neurological deficits and death before distant spread of tumor occurs, suggesting that regional therapy has the potential of being successful. Furthermore, the pharmacologically privileged status of the CNS may be advantageous if it retards immune inactivation of the therapeutic agent, permitting the agent to have its effects on the far side of the blood-brain and blood-tumor barriers, but reducing systemic toxicity via binding of the agent by neutralizing antibodies when it reaches the blood. These potential advantages of regional therapy for CNS tumors have stimulated the examination of approaches for treatment of them by using regional approaches for delivery and distribution of the immunotoxin.

The delivery approaches cited above have been developed to increase delivery of macromolecules to the solid contrast-enhancing portion of brain tumors and to overcome the relative inaccessibility to therapy of the glioma cells infiltrating the brain. Injection into the CSF also has been investigated for treatment of neoplastic cells circulating in the CSF or lining the CSF spaces (leptomeningeal cancer). The development of a successful therapeutic strategy for regional therapy requires understanding of the advantages and limitations of these approaches. Since the issues that must be addressed for tumor targeting, drug delivery, and toxicity differ for the two general categories of tumor, leptomeningeal cancer and solid tumors, we address separately the therapeutic strategies for them.

4 Leptomeningeal Cancer

Meningeal carcinomatosis occurs in 5%–20% of all cancer patients, most of whom have either breast or lung carcinoma. As patients survive longer with improved systemic therapy the incidence increases. Further, in many patients leptomeningeal metastases develop when the systemic disease is stable. Spread via the CSF of certain primary CNS tumors, especially those that tend to occur in children, such as medulloblastomas and ependymomas, is also a common occurrence. Because of the perception of easily overcoming the problems associated with delivery of macromolecules to tumors in the subarachnoid space, immunotoxin therapy of CNS tumors began with investigation of treatment of leptomeningeal cancer.

4.1 Preclinical Pharmacokinetics of Immunotoxins After Intrathecal Delivery

Since the flow of CSF within the neuroaxis is unidirectional – from the ventricular system through the aqueducts of the brain into the cisterna magna, the spinal CSF, and over the cerebral convexity to be absorbed by the arachnoidal granulations into the blood in the saggital sinus – reliable distribution of drugs in the CSF requires that they are delivered into the ventricular system, rather than into the lumbar CSF. Investigations of the distribution of immunotoxins after intraventricular injection in nonhuman primates demonstrate reproducible distribution and predictable concentrations of the immunotoxin through the CSF space. When monoclonal antibodies specific for the human transferrin receptor (454A12) were conjugated to recombinant ricin A-chain 454A12-rRA and injected into the ventricular system of rhesus monkeys, the clearance of the conjugate from the CSF was about twofold greater than the rate of bulk flow of CSF. Since the conjugate was not degraded in the CSF, losses additional to bulk flow were attributed to diffusion into brain and transcapillary permeation (MURASZKO et al., 1993).

4.2 Preclinical Toxicity and Efficacy of Intrathecal Immunotoxin Administration/Antitumor Activity

Neurotoxicity of immunotoxins can occur through receptor-mediated uptake, when the receptor is expressed on normal, nonmalignant cells. As transferrin receptor exists in normal brain the toxicity must be carefully examined. After delivery into the rat CSF, a monoclonal antibody (OX26) specific for the rat transferrin receptor linked to ricin A-chain was seven times more toxic than a monoclonal antibody specific to the human transferrin receptor (454A12) linked to ricin A-chain. Thus, targeting endogeneous transferrin receptors appears to produce toxicity. Fortunately, human transferrin binds to mouse, rat, monkey, and human transferrin receptors with similar affinity. Thus, toxicity of Tfn-CRM107 to normal brain, via

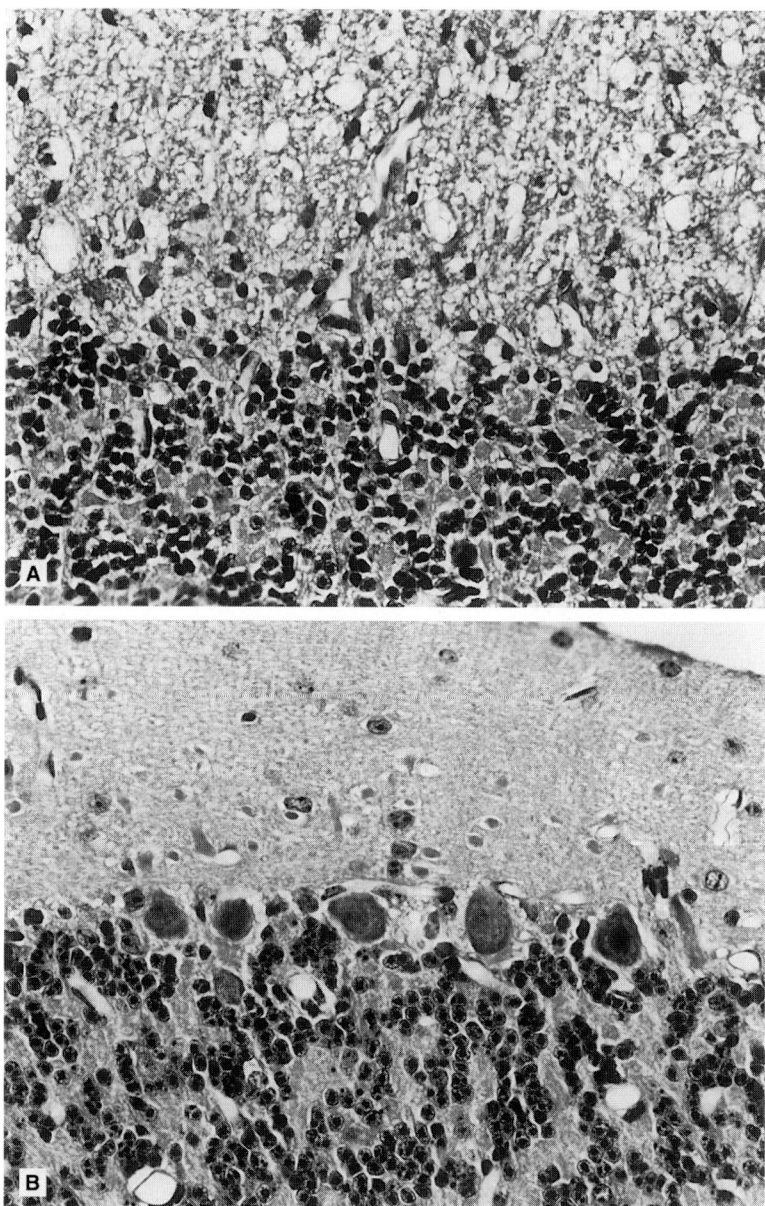

Fig. 1A,B. Purkinje cell loss after intrathecal administration of **A** immunotoxin 454A12-rRA at a nominal CSF concemtration of 1.8×10^{-6}M compared to **B** saline control

the targeting agent, can be accurately assessed in animals. This is in contrast to monoclonal antibodies and single chain immunotoxins, in which the mouse anti-human antigen antibodies often do not cross-react with the comparable antigen in rodents. For these reasons the toxicity of most immunotoxins has been difficult to determine prior to human trials.

Neurotoxicity of immunotoxins can also occur through nonspecific, nonreceptor-mediated uptake by cells. The key to the targeted toxin approach is that the receptor-specific pathway is much more efficient than the nonspecific uptake. However, in efforts to overcome the problem of access to brain tumor cells, doses of immunotoxins are often increased to the point where nonspecific toxicity occurs. Dose-limiting toxicity after injection of 454A12-rRA into the CSF is neurological. In experimental animals (rats and monkeys) it is a result of selective elimination of Purkinje cells (Fig. 1) and is associated with ataxia and lack of coordination. These histological and behavioral changes are dose-related and in monkeys occur at concentrations of 3.9×10^{-7}M or greater, concentrations that are several log higher (1000–10,000) than required for in vitro antitumor acitivity against many human cancers (JOHNSON et al. 1989). Immunotoxins made with CRM107 and saporin, targeted to a number of different receptors, also selectively kill Purkinje cells (BOOK et al. 1995; MURASZKO et al. 1993; RIEDEL et al. 1990; WAITE et al. 1995). In these cases, immunotoxin uptake appears to be through a fluid phase system and perhaps the large surface area and proximity of Purkinje cell dendrites to the CSF contributes to the high sensitivity of these cells.

To explore efficacy of immunotoxins for leptomeningeal carcinomatosis, a syngeneic animal model of leptomeningeal leukemia was developed in guinea pigs (ZOVICKIAN and YOULE 1988). As few as 100 L2C leukemia cells injected into the cisterna magna resulted in 100% animal death by 23 days and, the more cells that are injected, the more rapid is the onset of symptoms. Immunotoxins injected into the cisterna magna were effective in selectively killing 99%–99.9% of tumor cells in vivo and were curative at the level of a 5 log kill in some animals. These promising preclinical studies of immunotoxins for leptomeningeal cancer prompted clinical investigation.

4.3 Clinical Investigation

To begin to examine the pharmacokinetics and toxicity of intraventricular injection of immunotoxins in general, and 454A12-rRA in particular, and to detect whether 454A12-rRA had antitumor activity, we studied eight patients with leptomeningeal cancer (LASKE et al. 1997a).

When 454A12-rRA was coinjected with 99mTc-DTPA (an extracellular marker with low capillary permeability that is cleared only by bulk flow of CSF) into the ventricular system of humans with leptomeningeal cancer, the volumes of distribution (V_d) of 454A12-rRA and 99mTc-DTPA were 5–58ml, significantly lower than the CSF volume (about 125ml in humans), indicating at least partial occlusion of the CSF flow by subarachnoid tumor. The antitransferrin receptor antibody linked to ricin A-chain was stable in CSF. Clearance of it from the CSF varied greatly among the patients, but the average clearance was about twofold faster than 99mTc-DTPA (Fig. 2), an observation consistent with the preclinical

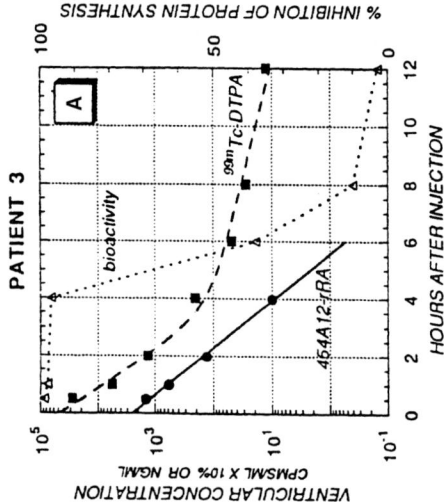
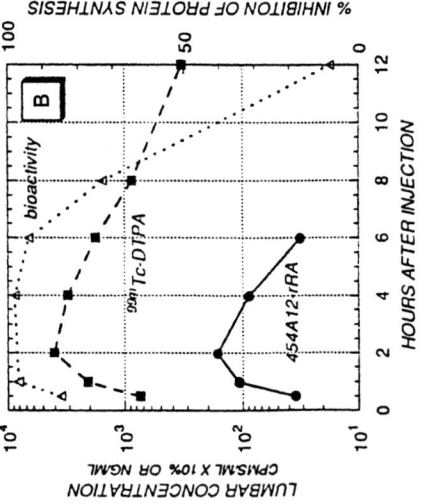
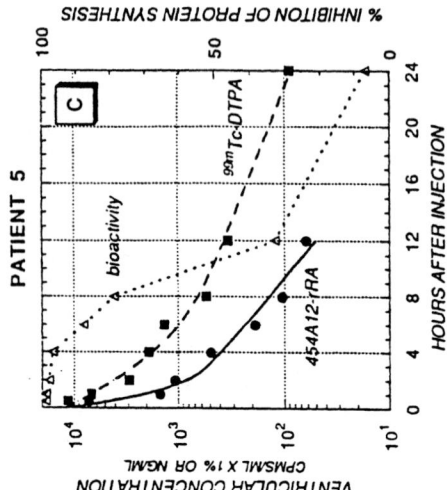
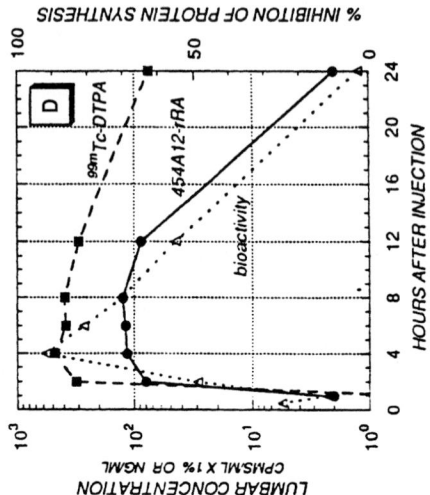

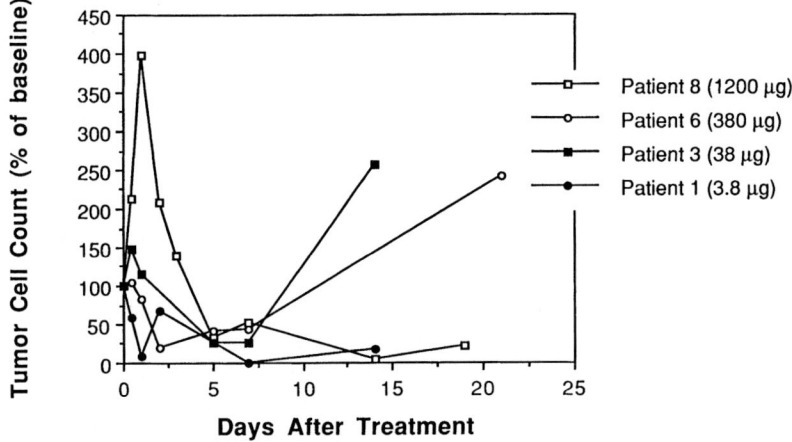

Fig. 3. Lumbar CSF tumor cell counts in four patients with leptomeningeal cancer before and after treatment with intrathecal 454A12-rRA. Counts represent the mean of three high power fields (hpf) counted for tumor cells after 4ml of lumbar CSF was filtered through a 5μm Millipore filter and are expressed as a percent of the baseline value before treatment

results in rhesus monkeys and, again, suggesting clearance by loss to brain tissue or across capillaries.

Toxicity was associated with, and seemed to be caused by, a CSF inflammatory response, which occurred at doses ≥ 120μg and became evident by the onset of headaches, vomiting, and altered mental status (LASKE et al. 1997). The syndrome was responsive to treatment with steroids and/or CSF drainage. No systemic toxicity was detected and no anti-conjugate antibodies were detected in the serum or CSF of any patient during 16 weeks of treatment.

In four of the eight patients a 50% drop in the tumor cell count in the lumbar CSF occurred within 5–7 days of the intraventricular injection of the immunotoxin (Fig. 3). However, clinical improvement occurred in only one patient, in none of the patients was the CSF cleared of tumor cells, and seven of the eight patients had MRI evidence of tumor progression within weeks of treatment. Since in several of the patients individual tumor nodules in the subarachnoid space around the spinal cord or in the paraventricular region were several millimeters in diameter, it is

◄───

Fig. 2A–D. CSF pharmacokinetics after intraventricular injection of a mixture of a conjugate of an antibody to the human transferrin receptor (454A12) and recombinant ricin A-chain (rRA) and ^{99m}Tc-DTPA, a marker that is only cleared from the CSF by bulk flow. CSF clearance after intraventricular administration of 38μg (patient 3, **A, B**) and 120μg (patient 5, **C, D**) of 454A12-rRA coinjected with 346μCi and 200μCi of ^{99m}Tc-DTPA, respectively. CSF samples were obtained from the Ommaya reservoir (**A, C**) and the lumbar drain (**B, D**), and assayed for radioactivity (*closed squares*), immunotoxin concentration by ELISA (*closed circles*), and bioactivity on K562 erythroleukemia Cells (*open triangles*). Exponential decay curves were fit to the ventricular data. The bioassays were conducted with patient CSF serially diluted tenfold. (From LASKE et al., in press)

unlikely that immunotoxin penetrated them to reach all tumor cells. It might be possible to overcome some of this difficulty with repeated treatment, permitting delivery of the immunotoxin deeper into the tumor by progressive reduction in the size of individual tumor nodules.

5 Parenchymal Tumor

Since most techniques of regional drug delivery (direct intratumoral injection, injection into a cerebral cavity after resection of a tumor, implantation of drug-containing polymers) depend on diffusion to distribute the drug in tumor and infiltrated brain, they achieve limited drug distribution, produce steep concentration gradients between the point of delivery and surrounding brain, and are sensitive to the molecular weight of the drug, factors which limit their application in research and in the clinic.

5.1 Pharmacokinetics of Convection-Enhanced Drug Delivery

In contrast to diffusion, bulk flow results from a pressure gradient; its flux is largely independent of molecular weight and with bulk flow the solutions distribute in relatively homogeneous concentrations (FENSTERMACHER and KAYE 1988; MARMAROU et al. 1984; ROSENBERG et al. 1980) We and our colleagues at the NIH explored the use of high-flow microinfusion to establish convective flow in the interstitial space of the brain for delivery and distribution of therapeutic agents of high and low molecular weight (BOBO et al. 1994; LASKE et al. 1997c; LIEBERMAN et al. 1995; MORRISON et al. 1994). Initially, BOBO et al. (1994) showed that convection-enhanced delivery enhances the distribution of sucrose (molecular weight 359 Daltons) and transferrin (molecular weight 80,000 Daltons) in the white matter of the cat brain by several orders of magnitude and achieves homogeneous distribution in the perfused region. In theory (MORRISON et al. 1994) and in practice (LIEBERMAN et al. 1995), even more uniform distributions occur in gray matter. The size and homogeneity of the distribution of ^{14}C-albumin in gray matter after convection-enhanced delivery in the cerebrum of rats were much greater than occurs even with small molecular weight drugs distributed by diffusion (LIEBERMAN et al. 1995). In primates β-dextran (10KDa) was distributed over more than 4cm of brain in a macaque after only 5h of infusion (LIEBERMAN et al. 1995), and the spread of labeled apotransferrin (MW 81KDa) was up to 3cm during an 87h infusion into the white matter of rhesus monkey brain (LASKE et al. 1997a), indicating the potential of convection-enhanced infusion to distribute macromolecules on a scale appropriate for the human brain.

Figure 4 compares theoretical penetration volumes achievable with delivery dominated by bulk flow to those achievable with delivery controlled by diffusion

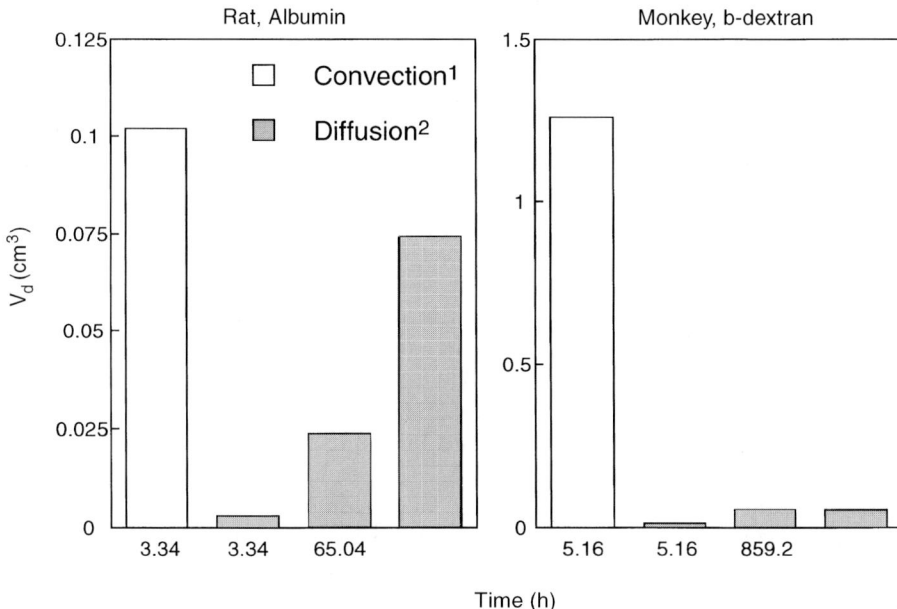

Fig. 4. Relative penetration volumes in gray matter after infusion utilizing bulk flow (convection) and diffusion. Volumes for convection are representative of the total tissue occupied by rat and monkey infusion volumes in homogeneous tissue; diffusion volumes are calculated for the same infusion time, the same infusion mass, and steady state diffusion. Note different Y-axis scales for rat (*left*) and monkey (*right*). For further details, see text. (From LIEBERMAN et al. 1995)

and shows that microinfusion that is dominated by convective transport allows the achievement of much greater penetration volumes than is obtained under conditions in which transport is dominated by diffusion (LIEBERMAN et al. 1995). Hypothetical volumes of distribution (V_d) for convection-dominated delivery were calculated that confine the infusate volume (20μl for the rat, 250μl for the monkey) to the gray matter. In Fig. 4, the open columns give the tissue volumes expected for convection-enhanced delivery using 0.1μl/min (rat) and 0.8μl/min (monkey) infusion rates. The shaded columns give volumes bounded by the locations where the interstitial concentration has declined to 10% of the infusate level. The first shaded column in each panel displays the diffusional volume predicted for the same time as used for bulk flow. These volumes are, respectively, 34-fold and 115-fold less than their 20μl and 250μl bulk flow counterparts. Furthermore, while the concentrations associated with diffusional delivery are computed to have declined tenfold over these distances, the interstitial concentrations associated with bulk flow remain nearly constant. In addition, the second and third shaded columns in each panel show that, while modest increases in penetration volume can be attained by greatly extending the infusion period of diffusion delivery, the maximum volume achievable by this approach is limited by the diffusional profile which develops at steady state and is less than the volumes achieved by bulk flow delivery in just 310min. In contrast, bulk flow penetration is limited only by the maximum allowable pumping pressure to the distance where spherical spread of the infusate has reduced the bulk flow velocity to that characteristic of diffusion. The tenfold greater bulk flow penetration volume predicted for the monkey relative to the rat in Fig. 4 largely reflects the ability to use a 12-fold greater infusion volume (250µl vs 20µl) in the primate without overflowing a gray-white boundary.

5.2 Preclinical Toxicity/Antitumor Activity

As discussed above, unlike many monoclonal antibodies, transferrin cross-reacts among species. Thus, the potential human toxicity of Tf-CRM107 can be evaluated in animal models. The toxicity of Tf-CRM107 injected intracerebrally was studied by stereotactically infusing 50µl of Tf-CRM107 solutions of increasing concentration (1.4×10^{-9}M to 1.4×10^{-6}M) into the white matter of the frontal lobe of rats (Laske et al., unpublished data). After repeated clinical assessment of the animals for 30 days, they were killed and the histology of the brain and systemic organs (liver, kidney and spleen) were examined to assess toxicity. The maximum tolerated dose (MTD), the highest dose that resulted in no animal deaths, was 1.67µg/kg Tf-CRM107 (infusate concentration, 7.0×10^{-8}M). An infusate concentration of 7.0×10^{-8}M also was the lowest infusate concentration at which histologic changes were noted in the brain. In one of the animals receiving this concentration, right frontal lobe encephalomalacia occurred. Histologic evidence of systemic organ damage did not occur until a dose of 33.4µg/kg was reached.

Since in vitro cytotoxicity of targeted protein toxins does not always correlate with in vivo efficacy or clinical applicability, we investigated the activity of Tf-CRM107 and 454A12MAB-rRA administered intratumorally against solid human gliomas (U251) in nude mice with established flank tumors (0.5–1.0cm diameter) (LASKE et al. 1994). The tumors were treated intratumorally with 10µg doses of Tf-CRM107, CRM107, 454A12MAB-rRA, 454A12, or buffered saline every 2 days for four doses. Tumor volume and animal weight were assessed every 2–4 days for 30 days after initiating therapy. With Tf-CRM107 tumor regression of > 95% occurred by day 14 in three of five mice, whereas treatment with CRM107 (the nontargeted toxin) alone produced nonspecific toxicity with death of all animals by day 10. At least a 50% decrease of tumor volume also occurred with 454A12MAB-rRA. In contrast, no regression occurred with 454A12 or control animals. At identical doses, Tf-CRM107 was more effective than 45412MAB-rRA in inducing tumor regression. In further testing the antitumor activity of TF-CRM107 was shown to be dose-dependent (LASKE et al. 1994).

These results demonstrated the in vivo efficacy of the targeted toxins Tf-CRM107 and 45412MAB-rRA against a human glioblastoma and suggested that Tf-CRM107 was the more potent agent. With regional administration, the effect of TF-CRM107 was tumor-specific and, in some animals, curative.

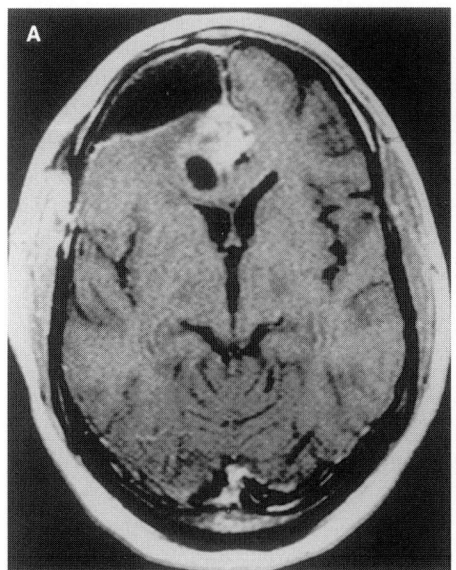
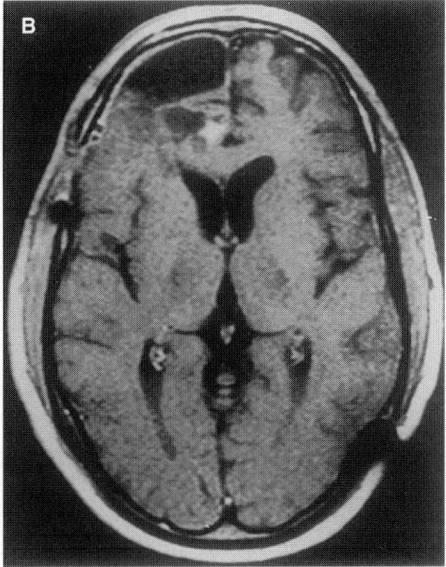

Fig. 5A,B. Gadolinium-enhanced T1-weighted axial magnetic resonance imaging (MRI) scans of patient 2, a 28 year old man with a right frontal anaplastic astrocytoma that progressed despite radiation therapy (6000cGy) and surgical debulking. Residual tumor posterior to the surgical resection cavity along the midline was rapidly enlarging immediately before treatment (**A**). Following three treatments of 0.1μg/ml Tf-CRM107 at doses (0.5, 2.0, and 2.0μg) well below toxic levels, tumor regression occurred within 3 months after beginning therapy (**B**). At 3 months, the patient was off steroids and had no neurological deficits. The time to tumor progression (MRI) was 10 months from the initiation of Tf-CRM107 therapy. (From LASKE et al. 1997b)

5.3 Clinical Trial

To evaluate the toxicity of Tf-CRM107 in brain when delivered by interstitial infusion in a dose-escalation schedule, examine the safety and utility of high-flow microinfusion in patients with intracerebral tumors, and determine if antitumor activity occurs at doses sparing brain injury, we performed a prospective trial of regional therapy with Tf-CRM107 delivered by high-flow microinfusion in 18 patients with malignant brain tumors refractory to conventional therapy (LASKE et al. 1997b). Ten patients had glioblastoma multiforme. To distribute Tf-CRM107 in tumor and areas of brain infiltrated with tumor, we used high-flow microinfusion to establish interstitial convection and enhance distribution of the macromolecule. Following a positive biopsy, one to three infusion catheters were placed with the tip at selected sites in the tumor using stereotactic guidance. The proximal end of the catheter was passed through the scalp and connected to a syringe pump and Tf-CRM107 was continuously infused into the tumor at 4–10μl/min. The initial Tf-CRM107 concentration (0.1μg/ml; 0.7nM) was 50-fold lower than the lowest concentration that caused histologic damage in the brain of rats after intracerebral infusion. It was escalated by 1/2 log increments every three to four patients at a given infusion volume.

Fifteen patients were evaluable for radiographic evidence of tumor regression. Following Tf-CRM107 infusion, at least a 50% decrease in tumor volume occurred in nine of the 15 evaluable patients (Figs. 5, 6). Reduction in tumor volume occurred no earlier than 1 month after completion of the first Tf-CRM107 infusion and the response did not peak in four patients until 6–14 months after the first treatment. Two patients had complete responses of the treated tumors. One had no evidence of tumor for 23 months after a single infusion of Tf-CRM107 into a progressing recurrent glioblastoma (Fig. 6). Biopsies of the region of treatment at 2 and 10 months after Tf-CRM107 infusion revealed inflammation and reactive changes, but no tumor cells. The second complete responder, who had a right frontal anaplastic astrocytoma, recurred in the infused region 5 months after treatment.

Tumor response appeared to be concentration- and dose-dependent. Only two of eight patients had partial responses in the first two treatments. In contrast, four of four patients treated with $\geq 1.0\mu g/ml$ had partial (2) or complete (2) responses. At intermediate concentrations, the responses correlated more with total dose than the concentration of drug; none of three tumors treated at $0.66\mu g/ml$ (total dose 26.4–$52.8\mu g$ during the first two treatments) regressed, whereas partial responses were achieved in three of three patients treated at $0.5\mu g/ml$, but with higher total volume and dose (total dose $60\mu g$ during the first two treatments). The mean pretreatment tumor volume in responders was less than that of nonresponders. The median survival after treatment in the group of nine responders who had malignant gliomas was 74 weeks (three of the responders were still alive 102–142 weeks after the first treatment) compared to 36 weeks for the nonresponders.

Intratumoral infusions of 5–180ml were well tolerated. There were no treatment-related deaths or life-threatening toxicity. There also was no irreversible toxicity associated with the interstitial infusion delivery technique. Although transient worsening of a neurologic deficit during infusion occurred three times in the 44 treatments, it was considered to be a result of increased cerebral edema, as it occurred only in patients with significant pretreatment edema and mass effect and the deficits resolved with steroid and hyperosmolar therapy or with completion of the infusion. Four patients with prior seizures had a seizure during infusion.

Fig. 6A–E. Gadolinium-enhanced T1-weighted coronal magnetic resonance imaging (MRI) scans of patient 10, a 48 year old woman with a right frontoparietal glioblastoma that recurred following surgical resection, radiation therapy (6000cGy) and chemotherapy (six cycles of BCNU, one cycle of procarbazine). This recurrent tumor was enlarging immediately before treatment (**A**). Following a 1 week continuous intratumoral infusion of $1.0\mu g/ml$ Tf-CRM107 ($27.3\mu g$ dose), there was an initial increase in the enhancing region 4 days after completing the infusion (**B**), which was resolving by 7 months after treatment (**C**). By 14 months a complete response occurred (**D**) and she was on no steroid medication. Her tumor showed no evidence (MRI) of recurrence for 23 months following the single Tf-CRM107 infusion. On the nonenhanced T1-weighted axial MRI images at 2 months (**E**), treatment-related changes adjacent to the treated tumor are evident as subcortical strips of high signal (*arrows*). Preexisting weakness of the left hand increased after completing the Tf-CRM107 infusion, but for 23 months she was otherwise neurologically intact. (From LASKE et al. 1997b)

Immunotoxins for Brain Tumor Therapy 111

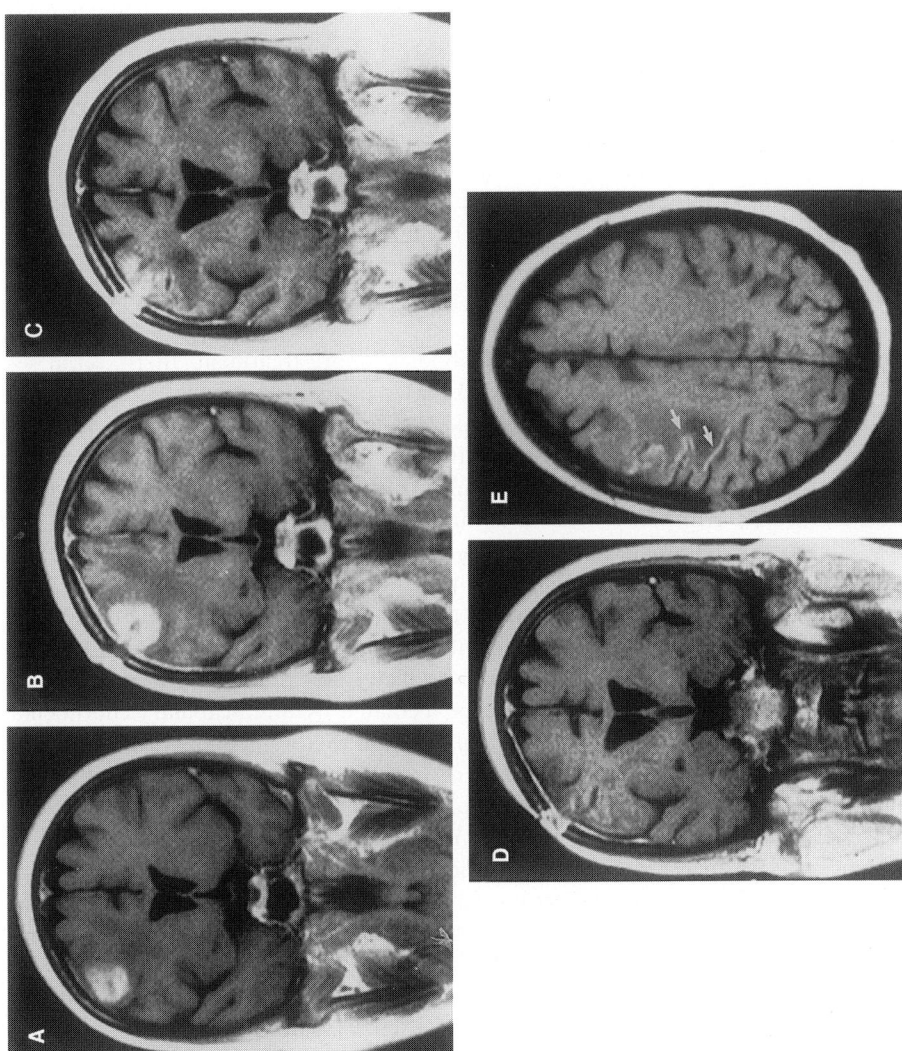

No peritumoral toxicity was detected in the eight patients who received 40ml of Tf-CRM107 ≤ 0.66µg/ml, although local toxicity occurred at the higher doses of Tf-CRM107. Peritumoral focal brain injury, which became apparent 2–4 weeks after treatment, occurred in all patients who received a concentration of Tf-CRM107 ≥ 1.0µg/ml. At 1.0µg/ml, all three patients had increased weakness (partial recovery occurred in two) associated with stereotypic MRI changes (serpentine strips of increased signal in peritumoral cortex evident on unenhanced T1-weighted MRI) that took up to 4 weeks after treatment to develop (Fig. 6). Stereotactic biopsy in these patients indicated that the MRI abnormalities were due to thrombosed cortical venules and/or capillaries.

No symptomatic systemic toxicity occurred. Transient elevation of serum transaminases (ALT, AST) occurred in 14 patients. Autopsy revealed no evidence of damage due to Tf-CRM107 in the five patients in whom the tissues outside the CNS, including the liver, were examined. Examination of the brain at autopsy in six patients revealed reactive changes in the white matter ipsilateral to tumor, consistent with chronic vasogenic edema and prior irradiation, but could not be related to Tf-CRM107 treatment.

All patients had anti-diphtheria antibodies before treatment. In 14, serial serum samples were obtained for > 4 weeks after the first treatment. In six of these 14, anti-diphtheria antibody titers increased at least twofold after treatment. This response did not correlate with Tf-CRM107 dose, steroid dose, or tumor response, and increases in titer after the first treatment did not appear to influence the likelihood of a tumor response with retreatment.

The results of the clinical trial demonstrated that regional therapy with genetically engineered protein toxins can elicit antitumor activity while limiting systemic drug exposure and toxicity. Even at the lowest doses tested in the clinical study partial tumor responses occurred without clinical or MRI evidence of toxicity to peritumoral brain, suggesting drug specificity for tumor. The dose-limiting toxicity, local brain injury, appeared to be mediated by brain capillary endothelial cell damage. Endothelial cells are the only cells in the brain to express significant levels of TfR. The extent of Tf-CRM107 distribution was not imaged in this study, but was inferred from the extent of the biologic effects. At the highest infused concentrations of Tf-CRM107 (≥ 1.0µg/ml), evidence of peritumoral injury was evident on MRI up to 4cm from the infusion point and tumor responses occurred in tumors 2–3cm in diameter, indicating that a therapeutic level of this large protein was distributed across several centimeters of tissue, and suggesting that this drug delivery technique has the potential of overcoming some of the problems imposed by the limited diffusion distance of drugs in solid tissues after direct injection.

To determine the response rate of interstitial infusion of Tf-CRM107 a larger phase II study that investigates more uniform dosing schemes and more stringent selection criteria, especially for tumor size, is underway.

References

Bergstrom M, Collins P, Ehrin E (1983) Discrepancies in brain tumor extent as shown by computed tomography and positron emission tomography using [^{68}Ga]EDTA, [^{11}C]glucose, and [^{11}C]methionine. J Comput Assist Tomogr 7:1062–1066

Bobo RH, Laske DW, Akbasak A, Morrison PF, Dedrick RL, Oldfield EH (1994) Convection-enhanced delivery of macromolecules in the brain. Proc Natl Acad Sci USA 91:2076–2080

Book A, Wiley R, Schweitzer J (1995) 192 IgG-saporin. Acta Neuropathol (Berl) 89:519–526

Boucher Y, Baxter L, Jain R (1990) Interstitial pressure gradients in tissue-isolated and subcutaneous tumors: implications for therapy. Cancer Res 50:4478–4484

Brem H, Piantadosi S, Burger PC, Walker M, Selker R, Vick NA, Black K, Sisti M, Brem S, Mohr G, Muller P, Morawetz R, Schold SC (1995) ÖPlacebo-controlled trial of safety and efficacy of intraoperative controlled delivery by biodegradable polymers of chemotherapy for recurrent gliomas. Lancet 345:1008–1012

Earnest F, Kelly PJ, Scheithauer BW, Kall BA, Cascino TL, Ehman RL, Forbes GS, Axley PL (1988) Cerebral astrocytomas: histopathologic correlation of MR and CT contrast enhancement with stereotactic biopsy. Radiology 166:823–827

Fenstermacher J, Kaye T (1988) Drug "diffusion" within the brain. Ann NY Acad Sci 531:29–39

Fishman RA, Chan PH (1990) Liposome entrapment of drugs and enzymes to enable passage across the blood-brain barrier. Pathophysiology of the blood-brain barrier. Elsevier Science, Amsterdam

Gatter K, Brown G, Trowbridge I, Woolston R-E, Mason D (1983) Transferrin receptors in human tissues: their distribution and possible clinical relevance. J Clin Pathol 36:539–545

Greenfield L, Johnson VG, Youle RJ (1987) Mutations in diphtheria toxin separate binding from entry and amplify immunotoxin selectivity. Science 238:536–539

Jeffries WA, Brandon MR, Hunt SV (1984) Transferrin receptor on endothelium of brain capillaries. Nature 312:162–163

Johnson VG, Wilson D, Greenfield L, Youle RJ (1988) The role of the diphtheria toxin receptor in cytosol translocation. J Biol Chem 263:1295–1300

Johnson VG, Wrobel C, Wilson D, Zovickian J, Greenfield L, Oldfield EH, Youle RJ (1989) Improved tumor-specific immunotoxins in the treatment of CNS and leptomeningeal neoplasia. J Neurosurg 70:240–248

Kalaria R, Sromek S, Grahovac I, Harik S (1992) Transferrin receptors of rat and human brain and cerebral microvessels and their status in Alzheimer's disease. Brain Res 585:87–93

Laird W, Groman N (1976) Isolation and characterization of tox mutants of corynebacteriophage beta. J Virol 19:220–227

Laske DW, Ilercil O, Akbasak A, Youle RJ, Oldfield EH (1994) Efficacy of direct intratumoral therapy with targeted protein toxins for solid human gliomas in nude mice. J Neurosurg 80:520–526

Laske D, Muraszko K, Oldfield E, DeVroom H, Sung C, Dedrick R, Simon T, Colendrea J, Copeland C, Katz D, Groves E, Greenfield L, Houston L, Youle R (1997a) Intrathecal immunotoxin therapy for leptomeningeal neoplasia. Neurosurgery (in press)

Laske D, Youle R, Oldfield E (1997b) Tumor regression with regional distribution of the targeted toxin Tf-CRM107 in patients with malignant brain tumors (in press)

Laske DW, Morrison PF, Lieberman D, Corthesy M, Reynolds J, Stewart-Henney P, Koong S, Cummins A, Paik C, Oldfield EH (1997c) Chronic interstitial infusion of protein to primate brain: determination of drug distribution and clearance with SPECT imaging. J Neurosurg (in press)

Lieberman DM, Laske DW, Morrison PF, Bankiewicz KS, Oldfield EH (1995) Convection-enhanced distribution of large molecules in gray matter during interstitial drug infusion. J Neurosurg 82:1021–1029

Marmarou A, Nakamura T, Tanaka K (1984) The kinetics of fluid movement through brain tiss. Semin Neurol 4:439–444

Martell L, Agrawal A, Ross D, Muraszko K (1993) Efficacy of transferrin receptor-targeted immunotoxins in brain tumor cell lines and pediatric brain tumors. Cancer Res 53:1348–1353

Morrison PF, Laske DW, Bobo H, Oldfield EH, Dedrick RL (1994) High-flow microinfusion: tissue penetration and pharmacodynamics. Am J Physiol 266(1,2):R292–305

Muraszko K, Sung C, Walbridge S, Greenfield L, Dedrick R, Oldfield E, Youle R (1993) Pharmacokinetics and toxicology of immunotoxins administered into the subarachnoid space in nonhuman primates and rodents. Cancer Res 53:3752–3757

Nicholls PJ, Johnson VG, Andrew SM, Hoogenboom HR, Raus JC, Youle RJ (1993) Characterization of single-chain antibody (sFv)-toxin fusion proteins produced in vitro in rabbit reticulocyte lysate. J Biol Chem 268:5302–5308

Pardridge WM (1990) Chimeric peptides as a vehicle for neuropharmaceutical delivery through the blood-brain barrier. Pathophysiology of the blood-brain barrier. Elsevier Science, Amsterdam

Pastan I, Willingham M, FitzGerald D (1986) Immunotoxins. Cell 47:641–644

Rapoport SI, Hori M, Klatzo I (1972) Testing of a hypothesis for osmotic opening of the blood-brain barrier. Am J Physiol 223:223–231

Recht L, Torres CO, Smith TW, Raso V, Griffin TW (1990) Transferrin receptor in normal and neoplastic brain tissue implications for brain tumor immunotherapy. J Neurosurg 72:941–945

Riedel CJ, Muraszko KM, Youle RJ (1990) Diphtheria toxin mutant selectively kills cerebellar Purkinje neurons. Proc Natl Acad Sci USA 87:5051–5055

Rosenberg FJ, Romano JJ, Shaw DD (1980) Metrizamide, iothalamate, and metrizoate: effects of internal carotid arterial injections on the blood-brain barrier of the rabbit. Invest Radiol 15[6 Suppl]:S275–279

Sevick E, Jain R (1989) Viscous resistance to blood flow in solid tumors: effect of hematocrit on intratumor blood viscosity. Cancer Res 49:3513–3519

Shin S-U, Friden P, Moran M et al. (1995) Transferrin-antibody fusion proteins are effective in brain targeting. PNAS 92:2820–2824

Sung C, Wilson D, Youle R (1991) Comparison of protein synthesis inhibition kinetics and cell killing induced by immunotoxins. J Biol Chem 266:14159–14162

Sung C, Dedrick R, Hall W, Johnson P, Youle R (1993) The spatial distribution of immunotoxins in solid tumors: assessment by quantitative autoradiography. Cancer Res 53:2092–2099

Trowbridge I, Lesley J, Schulte R (1982) Murine cell surface transferrin receptor: studies with an antireceptor monoclonal antibody. J Cell Physiol 112:403–410

Vitetta E, Fulton R, May R, Uhr J (1987) Redesigning nature's poisons to create anti-tumor reagents. Science 238:1098–1102

Waite JJ, Chen AD, Wardlow ML, Wiley RG, Lappi DA, Thal LJ (1995) 192 immunoglobulin G-saporin produces graded behavioral and biochemical changes accompanying the loss of cholinergic neurons of the basal forebrain and cerebellar Purkinje cells. Neuroscience 65:463–476

Youle R (1991) Mutations in diphtheria toxin to improve immunotoxin selectivity and understand toxin entry into cells. Semin Cell Biol 2:39–45

Zovickian J, Youle RJ (1988) Intrathecal immunotoxin therapy in an animal model of leptomeningeal neoplasia. J Neurosurg 68:767–774

Zovickian J, Johnson VG, Youle RJ (1987) Potent and specific killing of human malignant brain tumor cells by an anti-transferrin receptor antibody-ricin immunotoxin. J Neurosurg 66:850–861

Conclusions

A.E. Frankel and M.C. Willingham

1 Introduction 115
2 Dose-Limiting Toxicities of Targeted Toxins 115
3 Efficacy of Targeted Toxins 117
References 119

1 Introduction

The targeted toxin research reviewed in this volume includes recent advances in clinical applications of these compounds. The observation of clinical efficacy of both transferrin conjugated to mutant diphtheria toxin in high-grade gliomas and truncated diphtheria toxin fused to interleukin-2 in cutaneous T cell lymphomas and psoriasis are achievements for which all the members of the targeted toxin research community can be proud. The participation of so many colleagues in this field in this book has been a reflection both of the kindness and friendliness of the individuals as well as their commitment to working together to develop a new class of human therapeutics.

Rather than summarize the work of each chapter, several themes in clinical targeted toxin research are selected for discussion and postulation of possible avenues of further effort. These are not inclusive, but serve to show examples of how clinical observations may trigger new drug design and pharmacology.

2 Dose-Limiting Toxicities of Targeted Toxins

A number of targeted toxin trials have yielded unexpected normal tissue toxicities due to cross-reactivity of the tumor-selective ligand with normal tissue receptors (Table 1). In each case, cross-reactive antigen was also observed on normal tissues

---

Hollings Cancer Center, 171 Ashley Avenue, Charleston, SC 29425-2850, USA

Table 1. Normal tissue dose-limiting toxicities observed in targeted toxin trials

Protein	Normal tissue reactivity	Toxicity	Reference
260F9-rA	Schwann cells	Peripheral neuropathy	GOULD et al. 1989
OVB3-PE	Pontine neurons	Encephalopathy	PAI et al. 1991
Anti-TfR-rA	Brain capillaries	Encephalopathy	BOOKMAN et al. 1990

of nonhuman primates, but administration of targeted toxin to these animals rarely predicted the observed human toxicity. Thus, the selection of appropriate ligands for targeted toxins appears to be dependent alone on specificity of frozen section immunostaining of human normal tissues. Broad normal tissue testing panels should include samples of central nervous system tissue as well as peripheral nerves. Using such an approach, tumor-selective ligands can still be found. Lymphoid differentiation antigens, idiotypic determinants on B and T cell receptors, myeloid growth factor receptors, and unique oncogene products produced by glioblastoma multiforme (EGFRIII) and breast carcinomas (Her2-neu) are examples of possible targets for these toxic proteins. In cases in which compartmental delivery is possible, such as infusional therapy of central nervous system tumors, the EGFR may be an excellent candidate even though the antigen is widely dispersed on systemic organs. Another lesson from these clinical studies is the need for slow dose escalation. Some of the neurological toxicities appeared only in a few of the patients at a given dose-level (PAI et al. 1991; BOOKMAN et al. 1990). Other neurological events appeared many weeks after infusion (GOULD et al. 1989).

All the targeted toxins tested to date have shown vascular leak syndrome or vascular endothelial damage as an important dose-limiting toxicity. Various toxins employed in these immunotoxins include ricin toxin A-chain, blocked ricin, pokeweed antiviral protein, saporin, *Pseudomonas* exotoxin, and *Diphtheria* toxin (SENDEROWICZ et al. 1997; GROSSBARD et al. 1992; UCKUN 1993; FALINI et al. 1992; PAI et al. 1996; STROM et al. 1994). In each case, vascular injury developed over several days and was associated with hypoalbuminemia, transient hypotension, edema, nausea, vomiting, fevers, myalgias, pulmonary edema, or aphasia. No specific treatment has been reported to alleviate the syndrome, but many patients receive diuretics and/or albumin at some point in their course. Steroids have not been shown reproducibly to prevent or ameliorate the toxicity. No specific cytokine has been identified in the circulation of these patients. Vitetta's group has suggested direct endothelial injury as the mechanism mediated by the protein synthesis inactivating enzyme function of the toxins (SOLER-ROBRIGUEZ et al. 1993). Several approaches has been proposed to reduce this serious side effect. Smaller fusion toxins with molecular weights much less than antibody-toxin conjugates have been used in hopes of reducing the time of vascular exposure (PASTAN 1997). Other possible approaches include modulation of the apoptotic threshold of the normal vascular endothelium by administration of amifostine or similar cytoprotectants (CAPIZZI 1996). Alternatively, one can screen novel toxins prior to conjugation to ligands to select for those with the least inherent toxicity to endothelium.

3 Efficacy of Targeted Toxins

Applied to broad groups of patients with various malignancies in phase I and II clinical trials, targeted toxins yield response rates of 25%–35% with response durations averaging months (FRANKEL et al. 1995). Within these reports, examples are presented of durable complete remissions lasting years. An important effort in targeted toxin clinical development is the identification of clinical settings in which these reagents are uniquely efficacious and for which there are no other treatment options. Several possible disease categories are beginning to be defined (Table 2). SENDEROWICZ et al. (1997) reported a durable complete remission in a patient with a post-kidney transplant chemotherapy refractory B cell lymphoma. The optimal treatment for post-transplant lymphomas unresponsive to reduced immunosuppression and antiviral treatment is undefined. Aggressive cytotoxic chemotherapy is associated with poor response durations and a high rate of morbidity and mortality from immunocompromised host infections. The anti-CD22-dgRTA was not myelosuppressive and corroborated the striking anti-tumor activity of monoclonal antibodies alone in this condition (FISCHER et al. 1991). T cell large granular lymphocyte (LGL) leukemia is a chronic debilitating disorder in which the malignant T cell clone suppresses myelopoiesis. Most cytotoxic agents fail to reduce the tumor burden and uniformly aggravate the neutropenia (LOUGHRAN 1993). Anti-CD7-dgRTA was able to selectively deplete the marrow leukemic population and was associated with improvements in neutrophil count and red blood cell counts in two patients (FRANKEL et al. 1997). Four patients with advanced stage cutaneous T cell lymphoma (CTCL) unresponsive to topical and systemic chemotherapies had durable partial or complete remissions to $DAB_{389}IL2$ (DUVIC et al. 1997). Patients with advanced tumor stage CTCL generally fare poorly, with minimal responses to topical nitrogen mustard, psoralen and UVA light (PUVA), electron beam radiotherapy or systemic chemotherapy (HOLLOWAY 1992). Thus, this group of patients may be ideally suited for a nonmyelosuppressive, systemic drug. Even partial resolution of disfiguring cutaneous lesions can dramatically improve their quality of life. Small (2–3cm) high-grade refractory gliomas responded well to intratumoral infusions of Tf-CRM107 (Chap. 7, this volume). Survival in excess of 70 weeks was observed, which appears to be an improvement over historical controls. Further, the targeted toxin treatment obviated the need for surgical removal of necrotic

Table 2. Diseases states with favorable targeted toxin therapeutic index

Disease	Targeted toxin	Reference
Post-transplant lymphoma	Anti-CD22-dgRTA	SENDEROWICZ et al. 1997
T cell LGL leukemia	Anti-CD7-dgRTA	FRANKEL et al. 1997
Small unifocal refractory GBM	Tf-CRM107	Chap. 7, this volume
CTCL stage IIB	$DAB_{389}IL2$	DUVIC et al. 1997 and Chap. 6, this volume

LGL, large granular lymphocyte; GBM, glioblastoma multiforme; CTCL, cutaneous T cell lymphoma.

tissue which is often the sequelae of radiosurgery. The relative sparing of white matter fiber tracts by the toxin conjugate compared with high linear energy transfer (LET) radiation may account for the reduction in morbidity. We anticipate the identification of further specific uses for individual targeted toxins as more extensive phase II clinical trials are performed with these drugs.

An alternative approach both to reduce toxicities and improve efficacy for targeted toxins may be combination therapy with cytotoxic drugs or radiation. Supra-additive cell killing with combinations of immunotoxins and cytotoxic drugs have been observed in a number of studies both in vitro and in vivo in several malignancies (UCKUN et al. 1987; O'CONNOR et al. 1995; GHETIE et al. 1994; LIDOR et al. 1993; WEIL-HILLMAN et al. 1987; PEARSON et al. 1989a,b; JANSEN et al. 1993; LIU et al. 1996). Anti-CD5-ricin plus anti-CD7-ricin combined with 4-hydroperoxy-cyclophosphamide on T-ALL cells (UCKUN et al. 1987), anti-CD19-blocked ricin and doxorubicin or etoposide on B-non-Hodgkin's lymphoma cells (O'CONNOR et al. 1995), anti-CD19-ricin A-chain plus anti-CD22-ricin A-chain combined with doxorubicin, cyclophosphamide or camptothecin on Burkitt's lymphoma cells (GHETIE et al. 1994), and anti-p43 epithelial antigen-recombinant ricin A-chain conjugate with thiotepa or cisplatin on ovarian carcinoma cells (LIDOR et al. 1993) showed synergistic in vitro cell cytotoxicity. In vivo anti-tumor benefit from combining immunotoxins with cytotoxic drugs was observed using anti-CD5-ricin with mafosfamid in lymphoma (WEIL-HILLMAN et al. 1987), anti-epithelial antigen-*Pseudomonas* exotoxin conjugate with cyclophosphamide in colon cancer (PEARSON et al. 1989a,b), anti-CD19-ricin A-chain plus anti-CD22-ricin A-chain with methotrexate, doxorubicin, cyclophosphamide or camptothecin in lymphoma (GHETIE et al. 1994), anti-CD19-pokeweed antiviral protein with cyclophosphamide for B cell ALL (JANSEN et al. 1993), and anti-CD19-blocked ricin combined with cyclophosphamide, cisplatin, etoposide or cyclophosphamide, vincristine, doxorubicin and etoposide for B cell lymphomas (LIU et al. 1996). Rigorous isobolographic analysis and molecular mechanism studies were only done with the ovarian cancer immunotoxin/alkylator combination (LIDOR et al. 1993). Only the study of Vitetta and colleagues evaluated schedule dependency, showing in their system that toxin treatment had to precede cytotoxic drug exposure or administration for synergy (GHETIE et al. 1994). Such a cell-specific modulator of drug resistance as suggested by these studies would be clinically useful in patients with refractory neoplasms. The toxicities associated with nonspecific inhibition of membrane transporters or anti-apoptotic proteins can be avoided. Since the modulator is targeted to tumor cells, the only normal tissue side effects anticipated will be due to vascular endothelial injury. Since conventional cytotoxic chemotherapy rarely causes vascular leak syndrome, the combination of lower doses of fusion toxin with cytotoxic drugs should avoid this complication and improve tumor selective killing. The lower doses in the setting of drug modulation should reduce this toxicity. Further, the degree of resistance modulation by toxins may be potentially greater than with small molecule transport inhibitors. Since the prognosis for patients with refractory malignancies is so poor, any significant improvement in radiochemotherapy response would be useful.

References

Bookman M, Godfrey S, Padavic K, Griffin T, Corda J, Hamilton T, Ozols R, Groves E (1990) Antitransferrin receptor immunotoxin (IT) therapy: phase I intraperitoneal (i.p.) Trial. Proc Am Soc Clin Oncol 9:187

Capizzi RL (1996) Amifostine: the preclinical basis for broad-spectrum selective cytoprotection of normal tissues from cytotoxic therapies. Semin Oncol 23:2–17

Duvic M, Cather J, Maize J, Frankel AE (1997) $DAB_{389}IL2$ diphtheria fusion toxin produces clinical responses in tumor stage cutaneous T cell lymphoma. Lancet (submitted)

Falini B, Bolognesi A, Flenghi L, Tazzari P, Broe M, Stein H, Durkop H, Aversa F, Corneli P, Pizzolo G, Barbabietola G, Sabattini E, Pileri S, Martelli M, Stirpe F (1992) Response of refractory Hodgkin's disease to monoclonal anti-CD30 immunotoxin. Lancet 339:1–5

Fischer A, Blanche S, Le Bidois J, Bordigoni P, Garnier J, Niaudet P (1991) Anti-B cell monoclonal antibodies in the treatment of severe B-cell lymphoproliferative syndrome following bone marrow and organ transplantation. N Engl J Med 324:1451–1456

Frankel AE, Tagge EP, Willingham MC (1995) Clinical trials of targeted toxins. Semin Cancer Biol 6:307–317

Frankel AE, Laver J, Willingham MC, Burns L, Kersey J, Vallera DA (1997) Therapy of patients with T-cell lymphomas using an anti-CD7 monoclonal antibody-ricin A chain immunotoxin. Leuk Lymph (in press)

Ghetie M, Tucker K, Richardson J, Uhr J, Vitetta E (1994) Eradication of minimal disease in severe combined immunodeficient mice with disseminated Daudi lymphoma using chemotherapy and an immunotoxin cocktail. Blood 84:702–707

Gould B, Borowitz M, Groves E, Carter P, Anthony D, Weiner J, Frankel A (1989) A phase I study of a continuous infusion anti-breast cancer immunotoxin: report of a targeted toxicity not predicted by animal studies. JNCI 81:774–781

Grossbard M, Freedman A, Ritz J, Coral F, Goldmacher V, Eliseo L, Spector N, Dear K, Lambert J, Blattler W, Taylor J, Nadler L (1992) Serotherapy of B-cell neoplasms with anti-B4-blocked ricin. A phase I trial of daily bolus infusion. Blood 79:576–582

Holloway KB (1992) Therapeutic alternatives in cutaneous T-cell lymphoma. J Am Acad Dermatol 27:367–378

Jansen B, Kersey J, Jaszcz W, Gunther R, Nguyen D, Chelstrom L, Tuelahlgren L, Uckun F (1993) Effective immunochemotherapy of human t(4;11) leukemia in mice with severe combined immunodeficiency (SCID) using B43 (anti-CD19)-pokeweed antiviral protein immunotoxin plus cyclophosphamide. Leukemia 7:290–297

Lidor Y, O'Briant K, Xu F, Hamilton T, Ozols R, Bast R (1993) Alkylating agents and immunotoxins exert synergistic cytotoxic activity against ovarian cancer cells. J Clin Invest 92:2440–2447

Liu C, Lambert J, Teicher B, Blattler W, O'Connor R (1996) Cure of multidrug-resistant human B-cell lymphoma xenografts by combinations of anti-B4-blocked ricin and chemotherapeutic drugs. Blood 87:3892–3898

Loughran TP (1993) Clonal diseases of large granular lymphocytes. Blood 82:1–14

O'Connor R, Liu C, Ferris C, Guild B, Teicher B, Corvi C, Liu Y, Arceci R, Goldmacher V, Lambert J, Blattler W (1995) Anti-B4-blocked ricin synergizes with doxorubicin and etoposide on multidrug-resistant and drug-sensitive tumors. Blood 86:4286–4294

Pai L, Bookman M, Ozols R, Young R, Smith J, Longo D, Gould B, Frankel A, McClay E, Howell S, Reed E, Willingham M, FitzGerald D, Pastan I (1991) Clinical evaluation of intraperitoneal Pseudomonas exotoxin immunoconjugate OVB3-PE in patients with ovarian cancer. J Clin Oncol 9:2095–2102

Pai LH, Wittes R, Setser A, Willingham MC, Pastan I (1996) Treatment of advanced solid tumors with immunotoxin LMB-1: an antibody linked to Pseudomonas exotoxin. Nature Med 2:350–353

Pastan IH (1997) Tumor immunotoxins: technology closes in on potential. Adv Oncol 13:3–9

Pearson J, FitzGerald D, Willingham M, Wiltrout R, Pastan I, Longo D (1989a) Chemoimmunotoxin therapy against a human colon tumor (HT-29) xenograft in nude mice. Cancer Res 49:3562–3567

Pearson J, Sivam G, Manger R, Wiltrout R, Morgan A, Longo D (1989b) Enhanced therapeutic efficacy of an immunotoxin in combination with chemotherapy against an intraperitoneal human tumor xenograft in athymic mice. Cancer Res 49:4990–4995

Senderowicz AM, Vitetta E, Headlee D, Ghetie V, Uhr JW, Figg WD, Lush RM, Stetler-Stevenson M, Kershaw G, Kingma DW, Jaffe ES, Sausville EA (1997) Complete sustained response of a refractory, post-transplantation, large B-cell lymphoma to an anti-CD22 immunotoxin. Ann Intern Med 126:882–885

Soler-Rodriguez A, Ghetie M, Oppenheimer-Marks N, Uhr J, Vitetta E (1993) Ricin A-chain and ricin A-chain immunotoxins rapidly damage human endothelial cells: implications for vascular leak syndrome. Exp Cell Res 206:227–234

Strom T, Kelley V, Murphy J, Nichols B, Woodworth T (1994) Interleukin-2 receptor-directed therapies: antibody- or cytokine-based targeting molecules. Adv Nephrol 23:347–356

Uckun FM (1993) Immunotoxins for the treatment of leukaemia. Br J Haematol 85:435–438

Uckun F, Gajl-Peczalska K, Myers D, Ramsay N, Kersey J, Colvin M, Vallera D (1987) Marrow purging in autologous bone marrow transplantation for T-lineage acute lymphoblastic leukemia: efficacy of ex vivo treatment with immunotoxins and 4-hydroperoxy-cyclophosphamide against fresh leukemic marrow progenitor cells. Blood 69:361–366

Weil-Hillman G, Uckun F, Manske J, Vallera D (1987) Combined immunochemotherapy of human solid tumors in nude mice. Cancer Res 47:579–585

Subject Index

A
abrin   2
acute lymphoblastic leukemia (ALL)   46, 47
ADP-ribosylate elongation factor 2   3
AIDS-related NHL   46
ALL (acute lymphoblastic leukemia)   46, 47
animal models   19
anti-B cell immunotoxins   21
anti-B4-bR   38, 41, 42, 44
anti-breast cancer immunotoxin   21
anti-CD6-bR   50
anti-immunotoxin antibodies   25
anti-My9 MoAb   48
anti-My9-bR   38, 48
anti-Tac(Fv)-PE38   92
anti-transferrin-PE   84
antitumor activity   88

B
bacterial toxin   14
blocked ricin immunotoxins   35–54
blood-brain barrier   99
bolus infusion   23
brain tumor therapy   97–112

C
cancer   88
carbohydrate antigen   86
CD6-bR   38
chronic lymphocytic leukemia (CLL)   46, 47, 67
continuous infusion   23
cross-linkers   15
cutaneous T cell lymphoma (CTCL)   50, 67, 117

D
DAB_{389} IL-2   69–77
DAB_{389} EGF   78
DAB_{486} IL-2 fusion protein   67, 68
diphtheria toxin   1, 64–66
– fusion proteins   63–79
– – construction   66
– mutant CRM107   97
disulfide stabilized Fv   6, 8
dose-limiting toxicities   115, 116

E
e23(dsFv)PE38   92
e23(Fv)-PE38   92
encephalopathy   85
epidermal growth factor (EGF)
– fusion protein   77
– receptor   78
erbB-2   92

F
Fab′-RTAs   17
furin   5

G
gelonin   2
N-glycosidase   3

H
Hodgkin's lymphoma   24
HTLV-1   67

I
IGF-1   93
IL-2   93
– fusion proteins   67
– receptor   67, 92
IL-4   93
IL-6   93
immunogenicity of LMB-1   90
immunotoxin(s)   1, 14
– cocktails   20
– anti-B cell   21
– anti-breast cancer   21
– blocked ricin   35–54
– new   25
– *Pseudomonas* exotoxin   83–95
– recombinant single-chain   90
– ricin A chain   13–27

immunotoxin(s)
– ricin-based 36
– saporin 57–60
– single-chain 92
inclusion bodies 7

L
leptomengial cancer 101
LMB-1
– clinical trial 87
– immunogenicity 90
LMB-7 91

M
minimal residual disease 27
MM (multiple myeloma) 47
monoclonal antibodies 14, 86
– MAb B3 (IgG$_{1k}$) 86
multiple myeloma (MM) 47

N
N901-bR 50–53
non-*Hodgkin's* lymphoma 41, 46, 67

O
ovarian cancer 84
OVB3 86
OVB3-PE 84, 85

P
parenchymal tumor 106
PE (*see Pseudomonas* exotoxin)
pharmacokinetics 42
plant toxin 14
pokeweed antiviral protein 2
post-transplant lymphoma 117
proteasome 6
protein disulfide isomerase 5
Pseudomonas aeruginosa 83
Pseudomonas exotoxin (PE) 1, 87
– immunotoxins 83–95
– PE38 87
– PE40 87
– recombinant forms 87
psoriasis 77

R
recombinant ricin A-chain 16
– clinical trials 20
recombinant single-chain immunotoxins 90
ricin 1
– A chain immunotoxins 13–27
– based immunotoxins 36

S
saporin immunotoxins 57–60
single chain
– Fv 8
– immunotoxin 92
small unifocal refractory GBM 117
SO6 57

T
T cell LGL leukemia 117
TGF-α 93
toxins 14
TP40 (TGFα-PE40) 93
transferrin receptor 98
translocation 2

U
urokinase 5

V
vascular
– leak syndrome 24, 94
– targeting 26

X
X-ray crystallography 830

Current Topics in Microbiology and Immunology

Volumes published since 1989 (and still available)

Vol. 194: **Potter, Michael; Melchers, Fritz (Eds.):** Mechanisms in B-cell Neoplasia. 1995. 152 figs. XXV, 458 pp. ISBN 3-540-58447-1

Vol. 195: **Montecucco, Cesare (Ed.):** Clostridial Neurotoxins. 1995. 28 figs. XI., 278 pp. ISBN 3-540-58452-8

Vol. 196: **Koprowski, Hilary; Maeda, Hiroshi (Eds.):** The Role of Nitric Oxide in Physiology and Pathophysiology. 1995. 21 figs. IX, 90 pp. ISBN 3-540-58214-2

Vol. 197: **Meyer, Peter (Ed.):** Gene Silencing in Higher Plants and Related Phenomena in Other Eukaryotes. 1995. 17 figs. IX, 232 pp. ISBN 3-540-58236-3

Vol. 198: **Griffiths, Gillian M.; Tschopp, Jürg (Eds.):** Pathways for Cytolysis. 1995. 45 figs. IX, 224 pp. ISBN 3-540-58725-X

Vol. 199/I: **Doerfler, Walter; Böhm, Petra (Eds.):** The Molecular Repertoire of Adenoviruses I. 1995. 51 figs. XIII, 280 pp. ISBN 3-540-58828-0

Vol. 199/II: **Doerfler, Walter; Böhm, Petra (Eds.):** The Molecular Repertoire of Adenoviruses II. 1995. 36 figs. XIII, 278 pp. ISBN 3-540-58829-9

Vol. 199/III: **Doerfler, Walter; Böhm, Petra (Eds.):** The Molecular Repertoire of Adenoviruses III. 1995. 51 figs. XIII, 310 pp. ISBN 3-540-58987-2

Vol. 200: **Kroemer, Guido; Martinez-A., Carlos (Eds.):** Apoptosis in Immunology. 1995. 14 figs. XI, 242 pp. ISBN 3-540-58756-X

Vol. 201: **Kosco-Vilbois, Marie H. (Ed.):** An Antigen Depository of the Immune System: Follicular Dendritic Cells. 1995. 39 figs. IX, 209 pp. ISBN 3-540-59013-7

Vol. 202: **Oldstone, Michael B. A.; Vitković, Ljubiša (Eds.):** HIV and Dementia. 1995. 40 figs. XIII, 279 pp. ISBN 3-540-59117-6

Vol. 203: **Sarnow, Peter (Ed.):** Cap-Independent Translation. 1995. 31 figs. XI, 183 pp. ISBN 3-540-59121-4

Vol. 204: **Saedler, Heinz; Gierl, Alfons (Eds.):** Transposable Elements. 1995. 42 figs. IX, 234 pp. ISBN 3-540-59342-X

Vol. 205: **Littman, Dan R. (Ed.):** The CD4 Molecule. 1995. 29 figs. XIII, 182 pp. ISBN 3-540-59344-6

Vol. 206: **Chisari, Francis V.; Oldstone, Michael B. A. (Eds.):** Transgenic Models of Human Viral and Immunological Disease. 1995. 53 figs. XI, 345 pp. ISBN 3-540-59341-1

Vol. 207: **Prusiner, Stanley B. (Ed.):** Prions Prions Prions. 1995. 42 figs. VII, 163 pp. ISBN 3-540-59343-8

Vol. 208: **Farnham, Peggy J. (Ed.):** Transcriptional Control of Cell Growth. 1995. 17 figs. IX, 141 pp. ISBN 3-540-60113-9

Vol. 209: **Miller, Virginia L. (Ed.):** Bacterial Invasiveness. 1996. 16 figs. IX, 115 pp. ISBN 3-540-60065-5

Vol. 210: **Potter, Michael; Rose, Noel R. (Eds.):** Immunology of Silicones. 1996. 136 figs. XX, 430 pp. ISBN 3-540-60272-0

Vol. 211: **Wolff, Linda; Perkins, Archibald S. (Eds.):** Molecular Aspects of Myeloid Stem Cell Development. 1996. 98 figs. XIV, 298 pp. ISBN 3-540-60414-6

Vol. 212: **Vainio, Olli; Imhof, Beat A. (Eds.):** Immunology and Developmental Biology of the Chicken. 1996. 43 figs. IX, 281 pp. ISBN 3-540-60585-1

Vol. 213/I: **Günthert, Ursula; Birchmeier, Walter (Eds.):** Attempts to Understand Metastasis Formation I. 1996. 35 figs. XV, 293 pp. ISBN 3-540-60680-7

Vol. 213/II: **Günthert, Ursula; Birchmeier, Walter (Eds.):** Attempts to Understand Metastasis Formation II. 1996. 33 figs. XV, 288 pp. ISBN 3-540-60681-5

Vol. 213/III: **Günthert, Ursula; Schlag, Peter M.; Birchmeier, Walter (Eds.):** Attempts to Understand Metastasis Formation III. 1996. 14 figs. XV, 262 pp. ISBN 3-540-60682-3

Vol. 214: **Kräusslich, Hans-Georg (Ed.):** Morphogenesis and Maturation of Retroviruses. 1996. 34 figs. XI, 344 pp. ISBN 3-540-60928-8

Vol. 215: **Shinnick, Thomas M. (Ed.):** Tuberculosis. 1996. 46 figs. XI, 307 pp. ISBN 3-540-60985-7

Vol. 216: **Rietschel, Ernst Th.; Wagner, Hermann (Eds.):** Pathology of Septic Shock. 1996. 34 figs. X, 321 pp. ISBN 3-540-61026-X

Vol. 217: **Jessberger, Rolf; Lieber, Michael R. (Eds.):** Molecular Analysis of DNA Rearrangements in the Immune System. 1996. 43 figs. IX, 224 pp. ISBN 3-540-61037-5

Vol. 218: **Berns, Kenneth I.; Giraud, Catherine (Eds.):** Adeno-Associated Virus (AAV) Vectors in Gene Therapy. 1996. 38 figs. IX,173 pp. ISBN 3-540-61076-6

Vol. 219: **Gross, Uwe (Ed.):** Toxoplasma gondii. 1996. 31 figs. XI, 274 pp. ISBN 3-540-61300-5

Vol. 220: **Rauscher, Frank J. III; Vogt, Peter K. (Eds.):** Chromosomal Translocations and Oncogenic Transcription Factors. 1997. 28 figs. XI, 166 pp. ISBN 3-540-61402-8

Vol. 221: **Kastan, Michael B. (Ed.):** Genetic Instability and Tumorigenesis. 1997. 12 figs.VII, 180 pp. ISBN 3-540-61518-0

Vol. 222: **Olding, Lars B. (Ed.):** Reproductive Immunology. 1997. 17 figs. XII, 219 pp. ISBN 3-540-61888-0

Vol. 223: **Tracy, S.; Chapman, N. M.; Mahy, B. W. J. (Eds.):** The Coxsackie B Viruses. 1997. 37 figs. VIII, 336 pp. ISBN 3-540-62390-6

Vol. 224: **Potter, Michael; Melchers, Fritz (Eds.):** C-Myc in B-Cell Neoplasia. 1997. 94 figs. XII, 291 pp. ISBN 3-540-62892-4

Vol. 225: **Vogt, Peter K.; Mahan, Michael J. (Eds.):** Bacterial Infection: Close Encounters at the Host Pathogen Interface. 1998. 15 figs. IX, 169 pp. ISBN 3-540-63260-3

Vol. 226: **Koprowski, Hilary; Weiner, David B. (Eds.):** DNA Vaccination/Genetic Vaccination. 1998. 31 figs. XVIII, 198 pp. ISBN 3-540-63392-8

Vol. 227: **Vogt, Peter K.; Reed, Steven I. (Eds.):** Cyclin Dependent Kinase (CDK) Inhibitors. 1998. 15 figs. XII, 169 pp. ISBN 3-540-63429-0

Vol. 228: **Pawson, Anthony I. (Ed.):** Protein Modules in Signal Transduction. 1998. 42 figs. IX, 368 pp. ISBN 3-540-63396-0

Vol. 229: **Kelsoe, Garnett; Flajnik, Martin (Eds.):** Somatic Diversification of Immune Responses. 1998. 38 figs. IX, 221 pp. ISBN 3-540-63608-0

Vol. 230: **Kärre, Klas; Colonna, Marco (Eds.):** Specificity, Function, and Development of NK Cells. 1998. 22 figs. IX, 248 pp. ISBN 3-540-63941-1

Vol. 231: **Holzmann, Bernhard; Wagner, Hermann (Eds.):** Leukocyte Integrins in the Immune System and Malignant Disease. 1998. 40 figs. XIII, 189 pp. ISBN 3-540-63609-9

Vol. 232: **Whitton, J. Lindsay (Ed.):** Antigen Presentation. 1998. 11 figs. IX, 244 pp. ISBN 3-540-63813-X

Vol. 233/I: **Tyler, Kenneth L.; Oldstone, Michael B. A. (Eds.):** Reoviruses I. 1998. 29 figs. XVIII, 223 pp. ISBN 3-540-63946-2

Vol. 233/II: **Tyler, Kenneth L.; Oldstone, Michael B. A. (Eds.):** Reoviruses II. 1998. 44 figs. XVI, 187 pp. ISBN 3-540-63947-0

Printing: Saladruck, Berlin
Binding: Buchbinderei Lüderitz & Bauer, Berlin